The SMART way

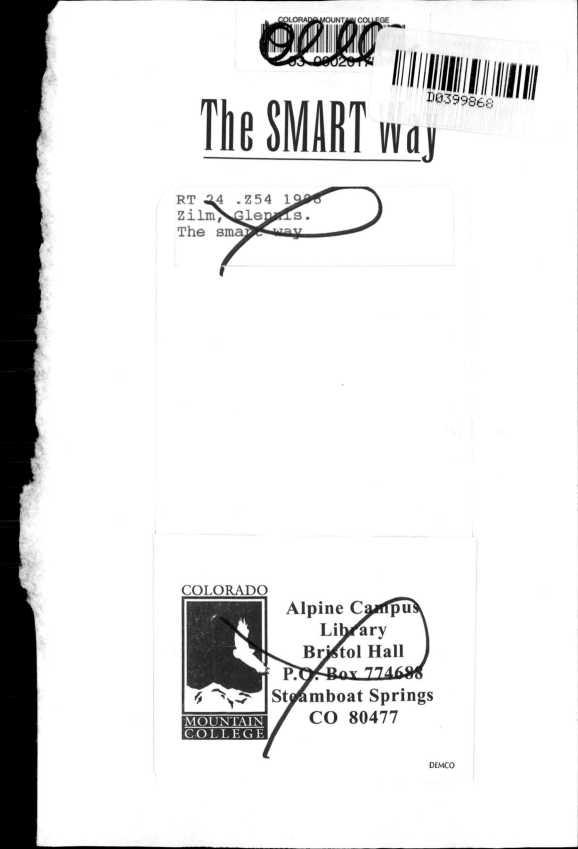

The SMART Way

AN INTRODUCTION TO WRITING FOR NURSES

GLENNIS ZILM

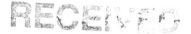

HARCOURT
BRACE
CANADA

Harcourt Brace & Company, Canada
Toronto Montreal Fort Worth New York Orlando
Philadelphia San Diego London Sydney Tokyo

Canadian Cataloguing in Publication Data

Zilm, Glennis
    The SMART way

Includes bibliographical references.
ISBN 0-7747-3563-5

1. Nursing – Authorship.   I. Title.
RT24.Z54 1998   808'.06661   C97–931602–2

Senior Developmental Editor: Laura Paterson Pratt
Production Co-ordinator: Shalini Babbar

Copy Editor: Dallas Harrison
Cover and Interior Design: Sonya V. Thursby/Opus House Inc.
Typesetting and Assembly: Carolyn Hutchings
Printing and Binding: Webcom Limited

This book was printed in Canada.

1 2 3 4 5   02 01 00 99 98

Preface

The purpose of good writing is to communicate ideas effectively — and effectively usually means as clearly and concisely as possible. Some writers forget this simple goal when they sit down to write. Others neglect this goal because they wish to impress readers with what they believe will be dramatic effects. The need for effective written communications in today's business world, including the health care system, has never been greater. Because of this, all nurses must be able to write well.

This book is intended to be a beginner's guide for nursing students who are having or believe they will have difficulties with written assignments. You probably have the ability to prepare academic papers, but you may have forgotten some of the rules you learned in high school. You may be at a different stage in the development of your writing skills and have different problems than your nursing classmates. For example, you may love to write and like to take a highly creative approach but find your instructors do not appreciate this. You may have taken several English courses already or may be taking writing courses concurrently with your nursing courses but find that some of the rules from these courses do not apply in nursing.

This small "how-to" book encourages you to write "The SMART Way." In Chapter 1, you examine the essential elements of communication — Source * Message * Audience * Route * Tone — and learn how to apply them. In Chapter 2, you learn about the writing PROCESS, a series of steps that help writers to organize content more easily and to write more quickly and effectively. Although the messages in these opening chapters may seem relatively simple, application of these skills can change your approach to writing and enable you to improve as a writer.

In Chapter 3, you review some common errors that nurses — and many other writers — make, and you learn how to avoid them. This book is not intended to replace a full-credit course in grammar and writing skills; it is intended to help high school graduates avoid errors that abound in academic and business writing. A few exercises scattered throughout the early chapters allow you to recognize problem areas in your own writing.

In Chapter 4, the focus is on references and bibliographies. You likely learned about them in high school, but they are much more important in the kind of writing you are expected to do for college and university papers. Lessons on the use of references and bibliographies are taught in many first-year, elective arts courses. If you have not taken such courses, this will be an essential chapter. Your nursing and science instructors usually expect you to have sound bibliographic skills and to develop them further with every paper you write. In this chapter, I also advise you of some valuable writing aids that you should have on hand and about how to use them.

Chapter 5 shows you how to apply the lessons from the first four chapters to term papers and written essays. The idea is to help you prepare better written assignments. In this section, I pay special attention to the style recommended by the American Psychological Association (APA). This is the most common style guide used in nursing schools and in nursing jobs following graduation.

The last chapter illustrates how you can use The SMART Way as a base for other written communications, such as letters, memos, résumés, reports, briefs, theses, articles, and research papers.

You should begin by going through the first four chapters carefully, doing the exercises as you go along. You can then turn to the sections that apply to the kind of writing you will be doing and see how the principles apply.

When you finish the book, you should be able to

- appreciate the value of written communications in professional development;

- understand the basics of written communications and appreciate the necessity of knowing the target audiences;
- recognize and select appropriate styles for written communications;
- prepare written communications with increased ease;
- recognize some of the common errors in writing and know how to avoid them;
- know how to use basic reference tools that assist writers; and
- write more effectively and get more positive results from written communications.

The SMART Way principles are based on insights I gained during master's studies in communications at Simon Fraser University. These insights were sharpened during workshops I gave for many years to registered nurses and others in the health care field. The workshop handouts eventually became manuals on writing skills for nursing students taking distance education nursing programs at the University of Victoria and the University of British Columbia.

Throughout the years, many talented individuals have assisted me in the development of the workshops, the distance education manuals, and this book. It is impossible to list them all. I owe a deep debt of gratitude to the hundreds of students who have been part of the evolution of this book. In particular, I have appreciated the help of the following colleagues: Pat Valentine, Ada Butler, and the late Jenniece Larsen, all of whom encouraged the development of the original workshops; Marilyn Willman, former director of the UBC School of Nursing; Barbara Courtney-Young and Shelley Lietaer of the University of Victoria School of Nursing; and Cheryl Entwistle of the UBC School of Nursing. I have also appreciated the comments and insights of the reviewers who critiqued the first draft of this book: Dale Rajacich, University of Windsor; Norma Wildeman, Wascana Institute; and Reida Woodside, University of New Brunswick.

I would especially like to thank the enthusiastic, supportive, persistent, and patient editors and staff at Harcourt Brace Canada, especially Kelly Cochrane, Laura Paterson Pratt, Marcel Chiera, and Sheila Barry, and in Vancouver Dallas Harrison.

Finally, I owe special thanks to my family for their patience, support, and encouragement during the last year.

Literally hundreds of students and health care professionals have used The SMART Way throughout the years and report that it has helped them to become better writers and communicators. I hope you, too, will find it useful in all your writing.

AUTHOR NOTE

Glennis Zilm is a freelance writer, editor, and writing consultant working in the health care field. One of her major interests is the history of nursing, and she is a co-author, with Ethel Warbinek, of *Legacy: History of Nursing Education at the University of British Columbia, 1919-1994* (Vancouver: UBC School of Nursing/UBC Press, 1994).

She has been the developmental editor for three nursing textbooks: *Canadian Nursing Faces the Future*, edited by Alice J. Baumgart and Jenniece Larsen (St. Louis: Mosby, 1988, 1992); *Nursing Management in Canada*, edited by Judith Hibberd and Mavis Kyle (Toronto: W.B. Saunders Canada, 1994); and *Community Nursing: Promoting Canadians' Health*, edited by Miriam J. Stewart (Toronto: W.B. Saunders, 1995). She has taught nursing and writing skills courses at the University of Victoria School of Nursing as a visiting lecturer, in both the distance education and the on-campus programs. She has been a consultant and occasional lecturer on writing skills for the University of Manitoba Faculty of Nursing and for the University of British Columbia School of Nursing.

A graduate of the UBC School of Nursing, she also has degrees in journalism and communications. She has combined her nursing background with journalism for more than 30 years. A former assistant editor of *The Canadian Nurse* and the former managing editor of the *B.C. Medical Journal*, she worked for five years with *The Canadian Press* in Edmonton and Ottawa, as well as in radio and television in Vancouver. She has been giving writing workshops to nurses and other health care professionals for 25 years.

Contents

APPENDIX A

Examples of APA Style for Full Citations in Reference Lists and Bibliographies 159

APPENDIX B

Sample Student Paper 169

APPENDIX C

Sample Business Communications for Nurses 175

APPENDIX D

Annotated Bibliography: Useful Readings/Reference Tools 185

1

The Five Elements of Communication

Written communications form a major part of the "glue" that helps people work together co-operatively and effectively. Written communications are vital in hospitals and other health agencies, and nurses must be able to write effectively. At one time, it was easier simply to talk to patients and colleagues; in modern agencies, writing (which includes messages such as e-mail) is often the only practical method of communication. Most staff nurses spend 15% to 20% of their work time writing. Nurse managers spend much more than that. Furthermore, as the interrelationships between hospitals and community-based care increase, written communications will likely increase in the future.

Because your nursing instructors know this, they want you to develop your writing skills, and almost all instructors in your academic courses base at least a portion of any assignment mark on writing skills. Good writing style also contributes to the mark for content; the writing must be clear (i.e., well organized and well expressed, with good grammar and punctuation) so the content of the paper will be clear. Unfortunately, most nursing programs do not include courses on how to write. You are expected to bring with you the basic skills you learned in high school; you may even be required to pass a college-entry examination to show that your writing skills are at that level. You are also expected to improve these skills as you complete your program. Usually, you must do this mainly through your own efforts. For this reason, many nursing students often opt to take electives in academic writing or in business English.

Some nursing courses focus on ways to improve your oral communication skills, especially in one-to-one communications (e.g., nurse-to-patient or nurse-to-nurse communications). Fortunately, the same *principles* of good oral communication also work in written communication.

The first step to good writing is to understand the five basic elements that affect all communications (oral, written, musical, visual, body language, and so on). I have organized these five elements using the acronym SMART.

The SMART Elements of Communication

Source
Message
Audience
Route
Tone

Understanding these elements of communication and their interrelationships will help you to

- recognize your strengths and work on your weaknesses;
- identify your objectives clearly and state your message explicitly;
- identify, understand, and respond to readers' needs;
- select the most appropriate method of communication (e.g., oral presentation, memo, letter, report, brief, review article, proposal, or whatever); and
- select the appropriate tone for the communication.

This breakdown of any single communication into these five basic elements may sound simple, but it really is not. $E=mc^2$ sounds simple, too, but that formula represents Einstein's theory of relativity! The important thing is that you understand the basic elements of communication.

The five elements fit together as a "package deal" in any communication; you cannot isolate any one element. Similarly, once you blend flour, sweetener, liquid, and fat, you cannot remove any one of them from the mixture. Yet those four basic recipe ingredients illustrate another factor related to communication principles. Those four ingredients are the basic elements of crepes, pancakes, scones, and pound cake; whether you get crepes or cakes depends on the relative amounts of those ingredients. Furthermore, you can vary the ingredients: you can use whole wheat flour, honey, skim milk, and oil, or you can use cake flour, white sugar, cream, and butter. The outcome will reflect the knowledge you have about the ingredients, how to mix them, how to cook them, and how to present them. The same applies in writing. So let us examine those five essential elements before we start to mix them.

■ Source

When you read a front-page newspaper headline that says "Student Fees to Increase," you immediately ask "Who says so?" If the source is some visiting pop star, you probably smile and treat the story somewhat lightly. If, however, the source for that comment is the president of your college or university, you begin to worry about having to pay more fees. You, the reader, are influenced by the source.

If you are leafing through a professional journal such as *The Canadian Nurse* and you see a title that applies to a nursing topic you have been asked to review, you should see who wrote the article by reading the author note, usually at the bottom of the page or at the end of the article. If the author is someone who works in the area, or if the remarks indicate the authors did research on the subject, this article may have more information about nursing methods than one written by a student or a non-nurse. Articles written by students or patients may still be valid, but you must weigh in your mind the qualifications and experiences of the source as it affects the content.

This need for readers to know the qualifications of the source of any communication should affect you as a writer. You need to weigh *your* qualifications for preparing the communication. Before you begin to write, you need to ask yourself "What are my qualifications for this communication?"

You may have experiences that give you knowledge about the subject. For example, if you are asked to write a paper on care of the elderly and you have lived for several years with elderly grandparents, you have some personal knowledge about problems people face as they grow older. If the topic for a paper is early human development and you have cared for small children, you have likely observed something about developmental stages that infants go through. If you are asked to write on environmental concerns and you had a summer job as a garbage collector, you will have practical knowledge about landfill sites and recycling habits. If you have diabetes, you bring a different perspective to a paper on this topic than if you have never known anyone with the condition. So you can draw on your lived experiences.

Furthermore, once you have had several classes on a subject and read the textbook, the instructor will expect you to have absorbed the basic concepts behind the course. If you have completed several nursing courses, you are expected to have more knowledge about anatomy, physiology, and health care needs than the average non-nurse. The latter will be true when you write papers for instructors in nursing; they soon expect a certain level of basic expertise based on all your courses. But does taking one course or reading a book make you an *expert* in the area? If you are not an expert (as will be the case when you are writing most student papers), then you may have to draw on the findings (research) of experts to bolster your statements or opinions. Where will you find the necessary expert opinions or facts — and how will you work them into your paper? To do this, you need to know how to use libraries to find information and how to use references in your papers so that your remarks are credible.

Sometimes you will have views of your own, even strong opinions, that should be included in your paper. In some assignments, your instructor will ask you to give your own views. However, you must still be able to substantiate them (give illustrations drawn from your experience) and expound on the reasons or rationales for your views. As well, you may need to show how your views compare with the "accepted wisdom" or traditional views in the area, and doing so may mean reading widely so that you can identify where your views agree with or differ from those of others. When you bring in supporting comments of others, you also have to judge whether the experts that you are using are accepted and whether they have done credible research.

You need to know other things about yourself as a source. As well as your knowledge of the subject, you need to know your strengths and weaknesses as a writer. Do you have good writing skills? Think about yourself as a writer. Can you identify your strengths and weaknesses? The statements in Exercise 1.1, which are based on comments by students in my writing skills workshops, may help you to identify some strengths and weaknesses. Think about each comment carefully and decide if it is a response that you might make. Would your classmates or other nurses make that remark? This exercise is mainly a self-assessment activity to tell you something about yourself as a source. However, it also provides some information about your audience.

In my workshops, about 65% of both student and graduate nurses indicate that they have difficulty expressing themselves. Surprisingly, most participants believe that others do *not* have this problem! You can take some solace in the thought that you are not alone — writing is hard work for most people. Almost everyone, even professional writers, dislikes writing and tends to put it off. Professional writers overcome this block by setting themselves deadlines and learning to stick to them.

Many people like to share their views, so this can be a real strength. Sharing your views will help you to get started with a writing project. Another strength that you may have identified in your self-assessment is that you like to read; this is an important strength for those taking

● EXERCISE 1.1 *Self-Assessment*

❑ I have difficulty expressing my thoughts.
❑ I dislike writing and put it off until the last minute.
❑ I like to share my views with others.
❑ I don't know how to find information on the topic.
❑ I like to read widely on a subject.
❑ I like to write.
❑ I cannot use a computer to write a paper.
❑ I have difficulty finding time to write.
❑ I like to write first thing in the morning (or late at night or other special time).
❑ I have difficulty getting started when I finally do sit down to write.
❑ I do not know the correct form that this written communication should take.
❑ I usually start working on an assignment the night before it is due.
❑ When I get started, I tend to be too wordy and too long.
❑ When I get started, I tend to be too blunt and too short.
❑ My writing is rambling and usually lacks a sense of focus.
❑ I have difficulty with basic grammar/spelling/punctuation.

postsecondary courses, because most instructors hand out massive reading lists. Reading the articles and textbooks required for the course is a splendid way to gather information.

If you identified as one of your strengths that you like to write, you are indeed a rare individual. (Even well-known novelists admit "I like being a writer — but I hate to write.") But do you only like to write about topics of your own choosing? Most of the "information writing" that you are required to do as a student or in the business world does not fall into this category. Often you must write what readers want or need to know rather than allow yourself to do "creative writing." This point is covered more fully in this chapter in the section on audience.

Finding information about a topic is always a problem. In your self-assessment as the source, determine your ability to use a library at the college or university level. Although you may have learned how to use the library in high school, you will find that there is an entirely different approach to library use at the postsecondary level. These libraries are much larger and are organized quite differently than most high school and public libraries.

About 40% of my workshop participants say that a major problem is finding time to write. This may be a bigger problem than you first anticipate. University and college courses often do not require large amounts of time in the classroom or lecture hall. However, much learning at the postsecondary level is expected to be self-directed; instructors expect that for every hour of classroom time a student should spend three additional hours in reading, writing, and thinking about (or discussing) course material. If finding time to write is your major problem, you may need a time management course rather than a writing course! Good writing takes time — even for professionals. You need to allow yourself time to write — and perhaps even to book "writing time" into your schedule. Consider doing so if you tend to leave the writing of an assignment until the night before it is due. Even if you are a superb writer, you usually cannot do a good job if you are rushed.

One small but important point to consider is the time of day that you like to write. Some people like to write first thing in the morning; if this is your style, then find a quiet room at home where you can write from 6 to 8 a.m. Others like to write in the evening. But doing so may be a problem if that is the time your family usually uses for family recreation. You may then need to move your workspace to another area of the house or plan to spend a couple of evenings a week working in a computer room on campus.

If you are a mature student, you may not know how to use a computer, but I strongly recommend that you learn as soon as possible. A computer or word processor — once you learn how to use it — makes writing and revising much easier. As well, some computer programs have aids, such as tools to check your grammar and spelling. It is highly unlikely that you can complete your nursing course without learning how to use a computer. Most students in your courses will be using computers to obtain information and to write their assignments, and if you do not know how to use a computer, you may find it difficult to keep up with these students. Many colleges and universities have computer rooms (sometimes in the library) where computers are available to students, so you can make use of one without having to spend a lot of money to buy your own. If you are not going to learn how to use a computer, then you should make arrangements to hire a typist who does use one. Although a few instructors will allow students to submit handwritten papers, most will require you to submit typed copies. Look for a typist who is good and quick (as well as inexpensive) and establish a good relationship with him or her. If you cannot type, you may end up relying on this person quite often. So in this self-assessment, weigh the information about your abilities with a computer carefully and decide if you need a computing course.

In my workshops, about 60% to 70% of participants believe that their writing is "long-winded" but that only about 30% of others have this problem. A much smaller number — about 10% — of participants believe that their writing is too blunt or too direct, or that they cannot make a letter, report, or assignment long enough. About 35% of participants say a major problem is that their writing is "too rambling" or that they cannot focus the message. And about 50% often find that the writing of others rambles — even in the articles assigned as required readings — and because of that the message is not clear to them. Almost everyone has difficulty in "getting started," although 66% of workshop participants do not envision others as having this common problem. A major reason why people come to writing workshops is to learn the correct format for a letter, report, article, or essay.

The final three remarks in Exercise 1.1 deal with actual writing problems (rather than with time management, for instance). You may need to think again about your skills in grammar, punctuation, and spelling. Usually, only 10% to 15% of participants at my workshops believe that they have difficulty with basic grammar and punctuation. However, when I mark papers from first-year nursing students, I find many serious errors in grammar and punctuation in most. A major reason for these mistakes is that the final draft of the paper was prepared in too much of a hurry — but these findings indicate that most students do not know themselves. About 80% of students admit that they have difficulty with spelling but that they do not own or use a dictionary. A dictionary is an essential tool for any writer. Computer spell checkers help, but you should have a good dictionary on hand as well. You should also know that business leaders and college/university instructors get upset about spelling errors in material that they have to read. Instructors, even if they, too, have difficulty with spelling, often take off marks for spelling errors in student papers; the rationale is that poor spelling or typing errors (called "typos") indicate a sloppy, rushed presentation. Problems with basic grammar, punctuation, and spelling are much more common than you may believe — and these problems can seriously affect your marks! Later in this chapter, there are some exercises that will help you to assess these areas.

■ Message

The second element in the SMART acronym is the message: the content of your communication, the information being conveyed. The message is the most important part of almost every communication. Because of this, you need to know exactly what your message is — and to know it *before* you begin to write. This means that you have to do a lot of thinking and planning before you begin to write. You need to have worked out in your mind what it is you want to say in your paper. This thinking process is the hardest part of writing.

Sometimes the topic to be covered will be given to you by the instructor. Sometimes you are asked to choose your own topic. Before you can begin to write, however, you really must identify what you want to say. You want your message in every written communication to be clear, concise, logically presented, accurate, well researched, and appropriate.

■ Audience

Just as it is important that you know and understand the source and the message, you need to know exactly to whom a communication is directed — the audience. If you are talking to a child who is your patient, you use different words and explain your points differently than if you are talking to a physician or nursing colleague. So when you sit down to write, you need to envision exactly who will receive your communication. Other textbooks talk about this person as the "receiver" or the "reader," but all experts agree that you need to think about the audience for your written communication.

Most student assignments are prepared for an audience of one person, the course instructor, so you have to consider the specific knowledge, skills, and expectations of that professor. This does not mean that you must kowtow to or play up to the teacher, just that you need to be aware of what your instructor has covered in class. For example, if you are aware that your nursing instructor supports one position and you are going to propose another view, you will need to anticipate the searching questions he or she would want answered. Do not assume, however, that your instructor knows what you mean; if you do, you may omit important pieces of the explanation. Remember, too, that instructors in psychology or law or anthropology might not be familiar with terms you use regularly in nursing courses; you may need to use a slightly different vocabulary in these courses than you would when writing for a nursing professor. Sometimes your instructor will ask you to write an assignment for a specific audience, such as a letter to the editor or an instruction guide for patients.

Furthermore, instructors in nursing courses frequently spell out clearly the points they wish you to cover in your assignments. Some state the style manual you must use or tell you the exact length of the paper. If so, you need to consider these points. If an instructor has told you what you are to cover in an assignment and you do not do this, you are going to lose marks.

If you are asked to write a book review, for example, the instructor may ask you to write it for specific readers. If the instructor does not specify the intended receivers, you may need to indicate in your review the audience *you* envisioned. For example, you might say: "This review is excellent for patients but does not contain enough detail for nurses."

■ Route

The route that you select to get your message across to the audience is also a vital element to consider, and it is often affected by the first three elements. The route, or "medium" as it was called by communications expert Marshall McLuhan, can vary considerably. For example, you can choose a song, a letter, a report, a play, a television show, a brief, a pamphlet, or a novel to send your message. These media will not be appreciated, however, if your instructor has requested a written essay of 2,000 words. There are even different kinds of written assignments (e.g., essay, review, report, article, personal journal). Most student papers fall into the general category of "essay."

Each route has its own format and therefore its own rules. For example, suppose you want to send a short written communication to a friend. Would you use flowered stationery, a business letterhead, a note card, a postcard? The "rules" vary for each different route. If it is a friendly, gossipy letter, you might like perfumed paper and purple ink — but they would not be appropriate if your friend works as a personnel officer and you are asking for an interview for a job.

You will likely have instruction in one of your nursing courses about the non-verbal messages you send when you are talking with someone. Non-verbal messages are conveyed by how you stand, by whether you smile as you talk, and even by what you wear (a business suit versus a party dress). You also send non-verbal clues about yourself and your written message when you choose items such as paper, cover folders, and type fonts for your assignments. If your assignment is handwritten on yellow paper with a dull pencil, then it conveys certain non-verbal messages to the audience — such as "This message was rushed and is not important."

The "rules" for the presentation of assignment papers at the college and university level are complicated. They are designed to make life easier for instructors who often must mark dozens, even hundreds, of papers each term. The rules are often so complex that there are whole books written about them. These books are called style manuals, and they are among the important writing tools that you should have on your desk.

Each nursing student should own a style manual. Although there are many good style manuals available, the *Publication Manual of the American Psychological Association* (American Psychological Association, 1994) is most commonly used in nursing programs. Other courses, such as English or biology, may call for other style manuals to be used, such as *A Manual for Writers of Term Papers, Theses, and Dissertations*, by Kate L. Turabian (1987), or *Scientific Style and Format: The CBE Manual for Authors, Editors, and Publishers*, by the Council of Biology Editors (1994). Some colleges produce a style guide that is recommended for their students when they begin their courses. You need to find out which manual is recommended for students in your nursing department and if this manual is acceptable for courses you may take through other departments.

All style manuals focus on details concerning the presentation of a written communication, such as what kind of paper to use, how wide to make the margins, or how to list each reference. Other details concern where to place your subheadings, when to use capital letters in the title of a book, how to punctuate when there are options, how to set up a table, when to use numerals and abbreviations (e.g., "10" versus "ten"; "hrs" versus "hours"), how to present quotations, and, most important, how to cite your references.

Most nursing instructors prefer the *Publication Manual of the American Psychological Association* — or APA *Manual*, as it is commonly called — because it is widely used for nursing publications. If you are planning to buy a copy, be sure to get the latest edition; do not get a second-hand copy of an earlier edition. By the time you graduate, you will be as familiar with this book as with a dictionary. In Chapter 4, I will review the main points of style you need for your early courses and describe how to use a manual.

Some instructors give detailed instructions on the style they expect you to follow. These instructions may be given on the assignment sheets for the course or in the course syllabus. These specific instructions from the instructor (your audience) override all others.

■ Tone

In addition to considering source, message, audience, and route, you need to consider the tone you will use as you write your message. Tone is influenced by all the other elements. It varies along a continuum from informal to formal. It also covers the emotional depth you wish to create as you write. For example, do you need to be dictatorial or coaxing? Do you wish to seem harsh and strident or pleasant and gracious? These represent variations in tone. You can be argumentative, persuasive, happy, sad, humorous, positive, negative, or sensitive depending on the words you choose and the way you arrange them.

Poet Robert Frost knew the importance of tone. He recognized that the inflection of a voice often meant more than words. If you word your sentences carefully, you can indicate inflections. An important factor in determining tone is learning to "listen with your mind's ear" as you write. If you "listen" to your sentences as you write, you will usually achieve the tone you wish to create, as in the following simple examples:

> He whispered, "Darling, I love you."
> "Darling," he growled, "I love you."
> "I love you, darling," he said.

The position of words within a sentence often helps to create emphasis and set the tone, as in the following:

> Inactivity, poor nutrition, and incontinence predispose patients to skin breakdown.
>
> Patients are predisposed to skin breakdown through inactivity, poor nutrition, and incontinence.

In the first example, listing the causes at the beginning of the sentence gives them greater impact. Depending on the purpose of the sentence within the rest of the paragraph, this positioning might be preferred. However, listing the causes at the end of the sentence gives them more emphasis and makes them more memorable, so this version may be preferred for an oral presentation.

Deciding what tone you need to use helps you to select words and phrases as you write. Consider the following:

> "Hey, dude, meet my old man!"
> "Joe, I'd like you to meet my husband."
> "Mr. Smith, I would like to introduce my husband."
> "Your Excellency, please allow me to present my spouse."

Tone creates personality in your paper. You can be bland and boring, or you can be exciting and refreshing.

Tone is affected by source, message, audience, and route, and you achieve it through your choice of words (vocabulary), as shown above. This choice includes the proper use of professional terms (e.g., "pain in the lower right quadrant of the abdomen" versus "tummyache").

Depending on the degree of formality required, you need to decide whether to use contractions (e.g., "isn't" versus "is not"). Most college papers are expected to be fairly formal in tone, so you would avoid using contractions, which are generally considered informal. Of course, if you are writing dialogue or quoting speech, you would include contractions to indicate that this portion of your paper is informal.

The use of first-person pronouns (I/we, my/our, mine/ours) also affects tone. In extremely formal presentations, writers refer to themselves in the third person (e.g., "Miss Smith regrets she cannot attend His Excellency's reception" versus "I am sorry that I cannot attend the reception," or "This author believes ..." rather than "I believe ...").

The use of first-person pronouns is permissible in formal writing today, although a few instructors (consider your audience) still prefer that you do not use them. For example, you should use "I" and the other first-person singular pronouns (1) when you are asked for a personal opinion or want to give one ("I think ..." or "I believe ...") or (2) when you have done the research or study and are reporting on it ("I found ..." or "In my study, ..."). When two of you have collaborated, the proper personal pronoun would be "we" (and the other plural pronouns). Usually, in your formal assignments, it is better to keep personal pronouns to a minimum and to keep yourself in the background — unless you are asked for a personal opinion.

First-person pronouns may be used in some kinds of informal writing when you want to establish links between the writer and the reader. These pronouns help to create a warm, personal tone and to establish a relationship with the reader, as in the following example:

In our hospital, we generally like to see nurses in white uniforms....

However, be sure that the informal tone is appropriate. Part of the problem with these pronouns is that readers are never quite certain who is meant. Does "we" in the sentence above refer to the writer and the reader? the hospital administration? patients? Consider the following sentence:

Nurses must take active roles in our society.

To whom does "our" refer: Canadian society? you and the instructor? Western society? nursing society? a specific association?

Finally, you also have to be careful of being *too* formal and avoiding the use of first-person pronouns altogether by referring to yourself as "the writer" or "this author." Such use can be confusing, as in this example:

These findings were reported by Baumgart (1988). This writer believes that....

Does "this writer" refer to the writer of the assignment or to Baumgart? Even the typeface (font) you choose to use on your computer can help to set tone. Pica and Times Roman typefaces (like this and similar to the one used for this text) are traditional but easy to read. Bold typefaces (**like this**) tend to be aggressive if used for complete sentences or paragraphs. Italic fonts (*like this*) are usually used in print to stress a word or phrase or to indicate a title. Some writers like to use an italic font in personal letters because it looks more like handwriting, but it is usually hard to read if used for a long passage. Some of the newer typefaces are fashionable but hard to read except in headlines. You have likely heard that the use of all capital letters in an e-mail message is referred to in computer jargon as "shouting."

■ More Self-Assessment

This chapter concludes with two more self-assessment exercises. They are designed to help you recognize your strengths and weaknesses, but the comment sections also provide information about style manuals and dictionaries that will likely be entirely new to you. After you have tried the exercises, go over the comment sections carefully.

If you have problems with Exercises 1.2 and 1.3, you need to own and reread a good basic text; I do not attempt to teach basic grammar and punctuation in this book. You probably do not need to take a complete course in English grammar, merely to review what you learned in school. Remember that if you make simple grammar and punctuation mistakes in a paper, no matter how excellent your content (message), you will receive a reduced mark! You, the source, are expected to have these basic writing skills.

● EXERCISE 1.2 *Punctuation*

1. The doctor of course writes the patients discharge order
2. We sent to the supply room for syringes needles and dressings for Dr Smiths special tray
3. Does the ward submit its budget by March 1st or March 31st
4. We shall never surrender was the closing line of one of Churchills best speeches
5. I want to go said Mary Will you go with me
6. Lets return to the ward said Mary so we can start the afternoon nourishments
7. The ladies coats were left in the hall but Johns coat was taken into the childrens bedroom

8. The boy said that he would be late and that we shouldnt wait for him we therefore left at five oclock
9. He wanted to go but his father said he couldnt
10. Three guests came George Smith chief of police John Jones chief librarian and Bob White assistant to the mayor

● COMMENTS ON EXERCISE 1.2 *Punctuation*

The level of skill needed to punctuate these sentences is equal to that of about Grade 6. You should, therefore, achieve an almost perfect score.

1. *The doctor, of course, writes the patient's discharge order.*
   Note that the commas go both before and after the interjected phrase. Do not forget the apostrophe. It must go before the *"s"* (otherwise, the last word would have to be "orders").

2. *We sent to the supply room for syringes, needles, and dressings for Dr. Smith's special tray.*
   Note that the comma after "needles" is *optional*; you were not wrong if you left it out. This comma, however, is a matter of style — and many style manuals, including the APA *Manual*, recommend that you place a comma before "and" in a series of three or more items (i.e., you would write "... apples, oranges, and bananas").

3. *Does the ward submit its budget by March 1st or March 31st?*
   This is an easy one — you need only put in the question mark. I hope that you did not put an apostrophe in "its" (making it into it's or, even worse, into its'). This misuse of its/it's is one of the most serious — and most common — spelling/grammar/punctuation errors that you can make!

4. *"We shall never surrender" was the closing line of one of Churchill's best speeches.*
   Note that you must *not* put a comma after "surrender." That would be the same kind of error as writing this sentence: The boy, runs. Should you use single or double quotation marks around the quoted portion of the sentence? This is sometimes a matter of style, but the correct usage here is double quotation marks.

5. "I want to go," said Mary. "Will you go with me?"

   There are other ways to punctuate here if you turn this into one complete sentence. However, the capital *W* in "Will" indicates that two sentences were used here.

6. "Let's return to the ward," said Mary, "so we can start the afternoon nourishments."

   Note the position of the punctuation in relation to the quotation marks. The first comma (after "ward") may be positioned outside the quotation marks (optional), so if you did this it was not incorrect. Some style manuals recommend that this comma be outside; the APA *Manual*, however, recommends that the comma be inside. The period here must be inside the quotation marks; this is not a question of style in this example. Note also that this was intended to be one sentence (differing from example 5).

7. The ladies' coats were left in the hall, but John's coat was taken into the children's bedroom.

   Use of the apostrophe to indicate possession is often difficult. If you have this problem, please review the rules in a good grammar book. Note that a comma is used before "but" in this sentence to separate the two independent clauses.

8. The boy said that he would be late and that we shouldn't wait for him; we therefore left at five o'clock.

   Style manuals recommend that, in formal papers, you avoid using contractions, such as "shouldn't" (for should not) or "I'll" (for I shall or I will) or "it's" (for it is). You must use them sometimes when you are reproducing speech, but otherwise you should avoid them in your written assignments. (I used the contraction in this exercise as a teaching point.)

9. He wanted to go, but his father said he couldn't.

   See the note on contractions for example 8. See also the note for example 7.

10. Three guests came: George Smith, chief of police; John Jones, chief librarian; and Bob White, assistant to the mayor.

    This is the best way to punctuate this sentence. The following punctuation would make the sentence difficult for readers to understand: "Three guests came: George Smith, chief of police,

John Jones, chief librarian, and Bob White, assistant to the mayor." Note that the comma before "and" here is not optional because it comes at the end of the interjected description of John Jones.

● EXERCISE 1.3 *Spelling*

Part A

Circle the *incorrect* spellings:

practice (verb)	practise (verb)
practice (noun)	practise (noun)
prenatal	pre-natal
paediatric	pediatric
analyze	analyse
dietitian	dietician
per cent	percent
labor	labour
focuses	focusses
program	programme

Part B

Read the following paragraph through just once, circling any spelling or typing errors:

This paragraph contains nine spelling errors of the type you are likely to run accross in your papers. Most errors are not in words like cholelithiasis or effervescent; such words set up immmediate warning signals, and you check them in a dicionary. Ordinary wards cause much more trouble; you barly give them a pasing glance — even those that everyone usually mispells. For this reason, editors advise that the finale step in proofreding is to read the text backward.

Count the errors you circled in the paragraph. If you did not find nine on the first reading, then go through it again more slowly looking for the errors and typos.

● COMMENTS ON EXERCISE 1.3 *Spelling*

Part A

In Part A, all spellings are correct *except* for practise (noun). The noun is always spelled practice. This part of the self-assessment exercise was meant to alert you to the fact that there may be more than one correct way to spell a word: spelling sometimes varies according to the preferred usage within a country.

For example, the generally preferred spellings in the United States, according to *Webster's Dictionary*, are honor, labor, harbor, color, program, analyze, criticize, percent, prenatal, postnatal, pediatric, fetus, dietitian, practice (verb *and* noun), center. In Britain, the preferred spellings, according to the *Oxford Dictionary*, of the same words are honour, labour, harbour, colour, programme, analyse, criticize, per cent (but percentage), pre-natal, post-natal, paediatric, foetus, dietitian, practise (verb), practice (noun), centre.

These are just a few of the many words that allow variations in spelling. Both dictionaries agree that the other spelling is correct and is permitted, but the one given first in the dictionary's listing represents the *preferred* spelling in that country.

Note that the spelling of focusses or focussed (where the final *s* of focus is doubled before the added *es* or *ed* endings) is the preferred spelling in Canada, according to the *Gage Canadian Dictionary*, but not in the United States or Great Britain. According to the lexicographers who put together the *Gage Canadian Dictionary*, Canada has adopted spellings from both the Americans and the British, with a few distinctly Canadian words and spellings.

Therefore, the commonly accepted and preferred usage in Canada of the words above is honor, labor (but the federal Department of Labour [a proper name] uses the *u*), harbor, color, program, analyze, criticize, percent, prenatal, postnatal, pediatric, fetus, dietitian, practise (verb), practice (noun), centre.

Dietician is an interesting word. The spelling with the *c* is acceptable but is going out of style; dietitian (with the *t*) is more common, and therefore preferred, according to all three dictionaries mentioned above.

Cigarette is another word that is changing; cigaret was used until the early 1990s in news stories in newspapers such as *The Globe and Mail*. The most recent style book for *The Globe and Mail* accepts the spelling as cigarette.

What does this mean for you, the student writer?

1. You need to be aware that there are some variations in spelling and that you need to pay attention to Source * Message * Audience * Route * Tone.

2. You need to own and use a good *college-level* dictionary (not just a cheap word book). The APA *Manual* advises that you should use *Webster's Dictionary*, but you (the source) can decide which dictionary you prefer for your university papers (provided you follow point 3 below). If, however, you are writing an article for publication in a journal, determine which dictionary would likely be the one most commonly used by its editors and readers (audience and route). For example, the *American Journal of Nursing* would use *Webster's*, and the British journal *Nursing Times* would use *Oxford*. I use *Gage Canadian Dictionary* because it gives preferred usage in Canada — but you need to have other dictionaries and be aware of some other differences if you wish to write for publication.

3. You must be consistent throughout the paper in your spelling. For example, you should not use "labor" on one page and "labour" on another. (Note, however, that when you are quoting from another writer and using quotation marks, you must keep the spelling used in the original — even if that spelling is incorrect, in which case you add [sic]). As well, if you are using a proper noun, you must spell it correctly (e.g., the Dieticians' Office at the Well Known Medical Center).

Part B

In Part B, you should have circled the following: accross immmediate dicionary wards barly pasing mispells finale proofreding. Two other comments on this exercise:

- "Backward" (rather than "backwards") is preferred usage in Canada (as is "toward," rather than "towards").

- A spell checker in a computer would not have picked up "wards" and "finale"; the *spellings* are correct, but in this context they are typing errors.

If you are having serious problems with basic grammar, review the section on writing skills in one of the books that help adults prepare for college-level entrance examinations. An exceptional book to help you assess your basic grammar, spelling, and punctuation is *How to Prepare for the GED High School Equivalency Examination: Canadian Edition* (see the reference list at the end of the chapter). Various editions are available, and you will likely find one in your local library. Two other superb texts for university students who have difficulty writing papers are *Making Sense in Psychology and the Life Sciences: A Student's Guide to Writing and Style (APA Format)*, by Margot Northey and Brian Timney, and *Fit to Print: The Canadian Student's Guide to Essay Writing*, by Joanne Buckley. Both contain good reviews of grammar. One of the most useful and most frequently recommended books for writers is rather old but remains a classic: *The Elements of Style* (3rd ed.), by William Strunk, Jr., and E. B. White.

You should start building a shelf of useful references to assist you in your writing. You need to own a good dictionary and an appropriate style manual. These two writing tools will be helpful in all your courses — and throughout your working life. I recommend *Gage Canadian Dictionary*, but *Webster's College Dictionary* is widely recommended in many schools of nursing in Canada; you may wish to inquire if your school has a preference. If you use a computer, you also need to know which dictionary is used in the spell checker that comes with your word processing software. The main thing about spelling when there are two acceptable choices is to be consistent throughout your paper. The APA *Manual* is the one most commonly used these days in nursing, and most instructors in other courses accept APA style. Note, however, that style manuals may offer different rules than some of the grammar books — especially about punctuation.

■ Summary

The SMART elements of communication — Source * Message * Audience * Route * Tone — form a "package deal" that will help you in your writing. Most problems that occur with your assignments come back to a consideration of one (or more) of these elements. Although they interact with one another and you cannot separate them in the finished version, you do have to consider each one carefully as you prepare your written communications. Once you get into the habit of examining your writing in the light of these five elements, you will improve your communications.

■ References and Recommended Readings

American Psychological Association. (1994). *Publication manual of the American Psychological Association* (4th ed.) Washington, DC: Author.

Avis, W. S., Drysdale, P. D., Gregg, R. J., Neufeldt, V. E, & Scargill, M. H. (1983). *Gage Canadian dictionary.* Toronto: Gage.

Buckley, J. (1995). *Fit to print: The Canadian student's guide to essay writing.* Toronto: Harcourt Brace.

Council of Biology Editors Style Manual Committee. (1994). *Scientific style and format: The CBE manual for authors, editors, and publishers* (6th ed.). Cambridge, UK: Cambridge University Press.

de Wolf, G. D., Gregg, R. J., Harris, B. P., & Scargill, M. H. (1997). *Gage Canadian dictionary* (rev.). Toronto: Gage.

McFarlane, J. A., & Clements, W. (1990). *The Globe and Mail style book.* Toronto: Info Globe.

Northey, M., & Timney, B. (1995). *Making sense in psychology and the life sciences: A student's guide to writing and style (APA format)* (2nd ed.). Toronto: University of Toronto Press.

Rockowitz, M., Brownstein, S. C., Hughes, A. S., & Peters, M. (1992). *How to prepare for the GED high school equivalency examination: Canadian edition.* Hauppauge, NY: Barron's Educational Series.

Strunk, W., Jr., & White, E. B. (1979). *The elements of style* (3rd ed.). New York: Macmillan.

The pocket Oxford dictionary of current English. (1978). Oxford, UK: Oxford University Press.

Turabian, K. L. (1987). *A manual for writers of term papers, theses, and dissertations* (5th ed.). Chicago: University of Chicago Press.

Webster's seventh new collegiate dictionary. (1965). Toronto: Thomas Allen & Son.

The Writing PROCESS

You are probably reading this text because you want to learn how to write more easily. You want to be able to write an excellent essay in one short sitting and avoid doing several drafts. Unfortunately, as dramatist Richard Sheridan said, "Easy writing's curst hard reading." As almost every professional writer will tell you, writing is hard work. Good writers usually go through several drafts so that readers can appreciate the results. However, if you understand the *process* involved in preparing a written communication, you will save time and effort and produce a better finished paper.

In this chapter, I provide some general hints on writing that will help you throughout your professional career and make some general comments on the use of libraries, which you will need to utilize in preparing your nursing assignments. I then describe the steps in the writing process using the acronym PROCESS.

■ General Hints

It is important that you have a good place to do your writing. You may do your best creative thinking in a big, soft armchair, sipping a coffee early in the morning before anyone else in the house is about. Or you may need to sit at a table in the library so that you can concentrate (and perhaps get away from noisy room-mates or children in the home). Or you may need a desk in a corner at home. Remember that going to university or college and writing papers *are* work! Give some thought to having a proper workplace.

You should also invest in some good tools, such as sharp pencils or good pens, erasers, good pads for drafts, good-quality, white typing paper (although not necessarily expensive, fancy paper) for the final draft, "white out," and good ribbons for your typewriter or printer. Later, I will discuss some of the other tools: a dictionary, a style manual, and a basic grammar reference. These tools are sound investments because you will use them in almost all your classes — and they will be helpful in the future when you need to write at work.

You should also have a personal bookshelf in your workspace and place the textbooks from all your courses there. Add copies of all the recent professional journals that you can gather, and keep them there throughout your courses; for example, if you have a friend who is a graduate nurse, he or she may be willing to lend you back issues of nursing journals. You should also have some files or boxes to contain articles that you photocopy. Articles copied for one paper often provide useful information in later courses.

If you are just starting your nursing program, you should learn to use a computer. Computer communications are here to stay and will be used much more frequently in the next decade than they are now. In the near future, nursing journals will likely be distributed electronically as "e-zines." Do not be discouraged about the technology. I learned to use a computer more than 15 years ago, when I was well into my forties, and computers in those days were not as user friendly as they are now! I recently learned to cope with e-mail and surf the Internet.

Computer programs can help you to improve your writing skills (and will help others, leaving you behind). You need to learn how to use them. For example, take time to learn what a spell checker will or will not do. A spell checker will not pick up typos. If you type

I was a nursing mayor at the University of New Brunswick

the spell checker will not point out that the word intended was "major." Most new computer programs also have a grammar checker. Many students will not use it because, when they try to check a long document, the grammar checker stops at almost every phrase and queries whether it should be fixed. It may then take you hours to identify which corrections are really necessary. Use the grammar checker on small portions of your writing, especially at first. It can be a valuable tool for learning your grammar. Some grammar checkers also give you information about the "reading level" (e.g., Grade 8 or Grade 12 reading level) and about the "fog index" (e.g., multisyllable words, passive voice, and long sentences) that make it difficult for readers to find your point. If your computer program offers these features, learn how to use them.

■ Using the Library

Assignments at the college and university level almost always require library research, so you need to be familiar with the libraries available to you. You can start with the library at your college or university, but do not neglect other libraries, such as a public library. You might also want to check other local hospitals and health agencies; some have excellent libraries for staff and may allow nursing students to use them. If you live in a city where the provincial nurses' association and provincial nurses' union are located, they also have useful library resources. Some provincial nurses' association libraries offer "distance services" if you join as a student member; the library will loan you books or even send you copies of relevant articles by mail or by fax. You need to check these services out and find out if there are charges for using them.

If you have computer access to the Internet, you can reach libraries from around the world. Most computer labs in colleges and universities have such connections, and it is often less expensive to do your Internet searches in these labs than on your personal computer at home. As soon as possible, check into the computer facilities available to you as a student.

Also spend some time in your college or university library finding out exactly what it offers and how to make good use of its services. These libraries usually offer orientation courses at the beginning of each term. Take the orientation course even if you think you are competent in the library. For example, college and university libraries usually have several computer or on-line catalogues, and you must know how to do a literature search or review using them. The basic catalogue provides information on the books available within the library; this catalogue is usually relatively simple, with a choice of "menu" items such as author or title. However, you can also search under subject headings, using keywords that help you to discover information on a topic even when you do not know the name of an author or the title of a book.

It is helpful to look for several articles on a subject in recent issues of professional journals rather than to read one or two books on that subject. Journal articles usually contain more up-to-date information than books. You will likely have been assigned one or two texts for the course, and they should form the base for your reading. As well, you should check out the topic in the texts for your other nursing courses, using the indexes to look for words that you think would provide information about the subject in which you are interested. You may also find reference lists within these textbooks that refer you to other information on your topic.

The reading list for your course may provide other good and relevant books and a few articles. However, spend some time finding out if there are even more recent articles on the specific subject in nursing or other relevant journals; keeping abreast of new articles always impresses an instructor! If you regularly spend time browsing in new journals or looking in indexes for journal articles, you will make faster progress. Early in your nursing program, you should spend some time browsing through the periodicals section of your library finding out which nursing, medical, and allied health journals are available there.

Most libraries also have access now to computerized indexes for journal articles; these indexes are often on separate terminals in one section of the library and are often arranged by general subject. For example, CINAHL stands for "Computerized Index to Nursing and Allied Health Literature" and is the one most useful for nursing students; MEDLINE focusses on medical and allied journals; and PsycINFO is an indexing service for psychology and allied disciplines. As well as on-line services, many college and university libraries subscribe to a number of CD-ROM services that index and provide access to articles in a number of journals. One CD-ROM service that you may find in many public libraries is the *Health Reference Center*; it provides selected indexes, abstracts, and, frequently, full-text articles from approximately 2,500 journals, including 150 core health journals (e.g., *Cancer, Journal of the American Medical Association*, and *RN*, to name just a few).

If your library has these indexing services or CD-ROMs, you can use keywords to prepare an up-to-date list of articles on your topic from hundreds of journals. In some instances, you can even print out the abstract or the complete article; most libraries require that you pay so much a page for them. Even if you cannot print out the articles, you can search for those in the journals in your library and read them there or copy them for later use when you write your paper. These articles can provide the background reading that you need for your topic.

Printing out or photocopying articles can be costly, but doing so may save you hours of work in the library. If you decide to photocopy articles or excerpts, be certain that you put the *full* bibliographic information on *each* document so that you will have this information for the reference list. This information includes

- full names of all authors;
- complete title of chapter or article;
- complete title of book or journal;
- full publishing details; and
- page numbers.

Full publishing information for journals or magazines includes the volume number and the issue number. These numbers may only be on the cover, masthead, or contents page and not on the bottom of each page of the article. Be sure that you get it *all*, because you will need it when you come to write your paper. Full publishing information for books includes the name(s) of the author(s) of the relevant chapter as well as of the editor(s) if the book has been compiled or edited. Use the title as it is printed on the title page (where it may differ slightly from the title on the cover of the book). The edition number is part of the title, so be sure that you note it as well. You also need the name of the publisher, the place of publication, and the year of publication; this information is often in small print on the copyright page (which is usually on the back of the title page). Write all of this information on each photocopy so that you have it there each time you need to refer to it. (There is much more about references in Chapter 4.)

As you do your library research, you begin to create a "working bibliography" or "working reference list" of articles and books for your paper. Many textbooks on writing suggest that you should do this on small file cards, and you may find this suggestion helpful. However, if you are using a computer, I recommend that you list your sources of information in a special file. If you do this, and make your notes on the computer, you will find that it is easy to integrate the references later into your paper. As well, you can combine your reference lists and refer to them again and again throughout your nursing program. Box

2.1 shows five references from a "working bib" that I developed when I was doing library research for a paper on tuberculosis (TB). The notes to myself include potentially useful quotations in the paper.

BOX 2.1 *Working Bib*

Working Bib for Paper on TB, August 1997:
Cohen, Felissa Lashley, & Durham, Jerry D. (1995). *Tuberculosis: A source book for nursing practice.* New York: Springer.

Available RNABC Library. Call number: WY 163 T827 1995.
The authors are both nurses and have written separately and together on HIV/AIDS. Cohen, a noted U.S. nursing author, is a professor in and the head of the Department of Medical-Surgical Nursing, College of Nursing, and the head of the medical-surgical department at University of Illinois Hospital, Chicago. Durham is at Indiana University School of Nursing, Indianapolis. As TB is once again on the rise, this book is a new student text after years when there were no nursing texts on the subject. An interesting quote from the book: "TB and HIV like to hang out together and they're a bad influence on each other" (p. 43).

Enarson, D. A., Grosset, J., Mwinga, A., Hershfield, E. S., O'Brien, R., Cole, S., & Reichman, L. (1995). The challenge of tuberculosis: Statements on global control and prevention (*Lancet* conference). *Lancet, 346,* 809-819.

Photocopy available GZ files.
"M. tuberculosis still accounts for more deaths world wide than any other single infectious agent" (p. 816). Article on global perspective.

Goldstone, Irene L. (1992). Trends in hospital utilization in AIDS care 1987-1991: Implications for palliative care. *Journal of Palliative Care, 8*(4), 22-29.

Photocopy available GZ files.
Nothing on TB, but relevant for current care of infectious diseases.

Grzybowski, Stefan, & Allen, Edward A. (1995). History and importance of scrofula (Department of Medical History). *Lancet, 346,* 1472-1474.

(continued)

Box 2.1 *(continued)*

Photocopy available GZ files.

A superb historical review of the history and causes of TB cervical adenitis (scrofula, from *M. bovis*); this disease may have provided immunity in its sufferers to pulmonary TB. Interesting closing paragraph:

> AIDS will open a new chapter in the story of scrofula. Not only can HIV itself cause lymphadenopathy, but also the loss of immunity allows for both the recrudescence of latent mycobacterial foci in the glands and the acquisition of new infections. (p. 1474)

Both authors are professors at UBC, and Grzybowski is Canada's foremost authority on TB in Indians and Inuit.

Houston, C. Stuart. (1991). *R. G. Ferguson: Crusader against tuberculosis* (Canadian Medical Lives Series No. 17). Toronto: Hannah & Dundern Press.

156 pp. Available Library of College of Physicians and Surgeons, Vancouver. Photocopy of pages 34-42 available GZ files.

Discusses formation of the Saskatchewan anti-TB league and various "firsts" that R. G. Ferguson instituted. For example, under his direction, Saskatchewan was the first area in North America to do an X-ray survey of the population and to conduct mass tuberculin testing on children and Natives (in Melville, I think. CHECK).

■ The Writing PROCESS

One of the biggest problems for every writer is getting started. Sometimes the problem is simply procrastination; you plan to write but keep putting it off until you are "organized." So you tidy the desk, make coffee, feed the goldfish, straighten the bookshelf, vacuum the living room, clean the stove, water the plants — and put off writing until the last possible moment (usually the evening before the paper is due to be handed in to the instructor!).

So how should you begin? You break down the big job into a series of separate steps, and then you take the first one. As American humorist and noted author Mark Twain once said, "The hardest part of writing is applying the seat of the pants to the seat of the chair."

Good writers go through several logical steps, and it may be helpful for you to devote some time to each of them. Dupuis and Wilson (1982), two excellent writing teachers, recommend that you use the POWER acronym. POWER stands for Plan*Organize*Write*Evaluate*Review. Their important point is that, if you want to have POW in your message, you need to *p*lan and *o*rganize before you begin to *w*rite. Markman, Markman, and Waddell (1994) say that there are *10 Steps in Writing the Research Paper* — and writing the first draft is step number seven! Back in 1971, Canadian author Pierre Berton said:

> It is not generally understood that most writing takes place away from the typewriter. When you finally approach the machine, it is already the beginning of the end. Nine-tenths of your work has already been done; it just remains to put on paper what you have already created. It is the creative process that takes most of the time. (as cited in Colombo, 1974, p. 52)

Figure 2.1 shows the various rungs that you must climb as you write your papers. Most student writers try to leap onto the ladder at the third rung; they plan just to sit down and write the assignment. You will have much greater success with your assignments if you deliberately spend some time on the ground and the first two rungs. Furthermore, you should make some specific deadlines for yourself. Do this as early as possible in the course. Read through your course syllabus and note the due dates for assignments. Begin right away to think about the first assignment and continue to think about it as you read the first lessons or attend the first lectures.

Spend the next few minutes really examining the ladder diagram. The arrow indicates that you may need to go back and forth! For example, you may plan to write on a certain topic, but when you get to the library to choose some readings, you find that nothing is available. So you need to step back and think about a new topic. Or, when you begin to organize your paper, you find that you need to go back and do further reading or thinking. An excellent idea is to note the date your assignment is due and then set a specific deadline for the first step.

RUNG 1: PLAN

In many assignments, your instructor will determine the topic for you. In some, you may choose your own topic. In either case, you need to sit and think before you sit and write! You even need to determine a possible topic before you begin to do any reading on it. If you spend a few minutes really thinking about your assignment, and sorting out in your mind the SMART elements of communication (Source * Message * Audience * Route * Tone) as they apply to the assignment, you will be much further ahead.

FIGURE 2.1 *The Writing Process*

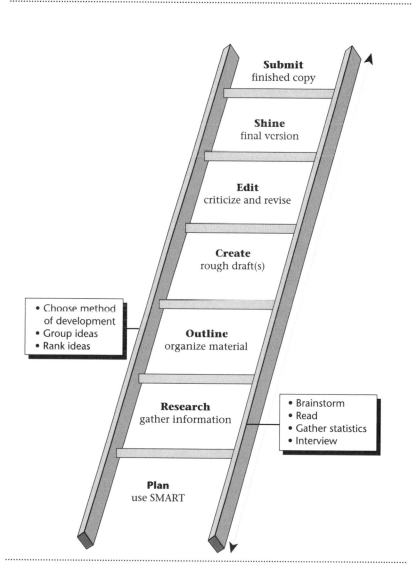

If you can choose your own topic, choose it carefully. Although it is a good idea to select a topic that you (source) like, you also need to select one that fits with the other four elements. Are you really knowledgeable about the topic, or will you have to do a great deal of background reading? Is the topic one that the instructor (audience) really asked for (or just one on which you want to write)? Think about your proposed topic (message) carefully. Is it too big to be covered in a paper of 10 pages or 2,000 words? If so, perhaps you should consider doing only one aspect of that topic. Is there enough information if you are asked to write a paper of 12 pages or 3,000 words? Can you get information on this topic, or are all the books on this subject likely to be out of the library already? Is this topic suitable for the type of assignment (route) you are asked to submit (book review, essay, personal journal, patient interview)? You may need to do some preliminary library research (see next step) before you can tell whether your proposed topic is feasible.

Think first of all about the audience (your instructor). Read the information about the assignment carefully. What has your instructor specifically asked for in the assignment? What has he or she told you about the topic in class? What references have been suggested in your course outline or in class as being pertinent to the topic? Think about the purpose the instructor has in mind in giving out the assignment. Is the purpose to see if you understand a point that was made in class or in some of the readings? Are you expected to answer a question in the paper? If it is the latter, is the answer to be based on reading or on personal experience? If you are to determine your own topic, ask yourself if your instructor is likely to be knowledgeable about that subject or whether you are more expert and will need to provide explanations.

This thinking/planning stage takes a bit of time, but it has two positive aspects. First, you can do it almost anywhere (riding home on the bus, waiting in the cafeteria for a friend). Second, it gets you started. And, if you like to be creative, it can be a highly stimulating time.

RUNG 2: RESEARCH (GATHER INFORMATION)

After thinking about the five SMART elements, as in Chapter 1, you will probably need to do some preliminary research before you can decide definitely on your topic and work out the plan for the next steps. For your first nursing assignments, usually this means doing some extra reading about what experts have said about the topic. In most courses, your instructors will give you lists of readings, and some of them may apply to your topic. However, you should do additional research by checking out the topic in a good library.

Once you have determined the topic, you can start to gather the information. You should also talk to others about the topic. Even chatting informally over coffee with fellow students might give you some ideas. Remember, you do not have to use these ideas if they do not fit with what *you*, the source, want to say. You might discuss the subject over dinner with non-nursing friends or family; you might be surprised to find that family members can suggest some good ideas! You can even use a computer to access the Internet and visit nursing chat rooms or networks to see what student nurses in other parts of the country have to say. As well as browsing on the Internet, you should certainly browse in a good library and begin your working bibliography as discussed earlier in this chapter.

RUNG 3: OUTLINE (ORGANIZE YOUR MESSAGE)

The next step on the ladder is to organize your information into an intelligent plan for communicating it in your paper. You may find it helpful to brainstorm. Sit down with a piece of paper and jot down (briefly, using only one or two words) all the ideas that you want to develop in the assignment. You might prefer to do this as a list, but others might like to do it as a "map" in which they put the central idea in the centre of a page and then group other ideas around it. When a subidea sparks other ideas, you group them around the subidea. The beginning of a map on the topic of flowers is shown in Figure 2.2.

Once you have come up with all the ideas that you want to put into your assignment, you need to organize them into some sort of order — you need an outline. You should remember the outline, because you learned about it in elementary school when you were first learning how to write essays. See Box 2.2.

You will remember that your elementary schoolteachers urged you to organize your papers into *three* main parts. This is still a good idea, although it will not work for all topics. Some topics need two parts, while some need four or more parts. The rationale behind this division into main parts, however, is that readers will be able to follow your thoughts. Keeping the main divisions to a manageable number (such as three) helps readers to grasp your ideas readily and to remember them easily. You may cover more than three ideas within a paper, but some of them will be organized as subparts of one of the three main ideas.

FIGURE 2.2 *Brainstorming Map*

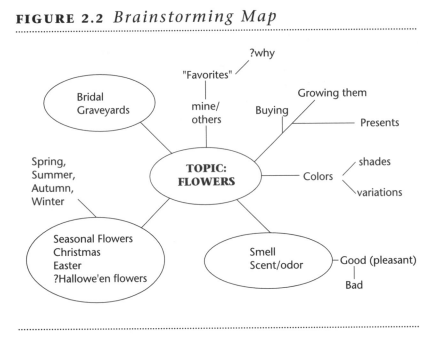

You also help your readers to understand your message by telling them in the introduction just what you are going to cover in the main part of the paper. And in the concluding section, you sum up your ideas briefly to remind the reader what was covered. In the journalistic

---

BOX 2.2 *Outline*

Outline
I. Introduction
II. Body
  A. First main idea
    1. Subidea to main idea
    2. Subidea to main idea
      a. sub-subidea
      b. sub-subidea
  B. Second main idea
    (and subideas organized as in A)
  C. Third main idea
    (and subideas organized as in A)
III. Conclusion

world, this organizational pattern is summed up this way:

- Tell them what you are going to tell them.
- Tell them.
- Tell them what you have told them.

This framework may sound rather simplistic, but you can still be creative within it. Remember that an assignment is not a mystery novel in which you save your point until the end of the book. Making your point clearly in the introduction will certainly help your instructor to understand what you are doing with your paper — and will likely pay off in marks!

Students who have major problems with written communications have failed to spend time on the three basic first steps of the ladder. Furthermore, these early steps are usually the fun part of writing. They represent the time when you can let your imagination flow.

You may want to finish the outline stage by jotting down several ideas for a title; doing so helps you to define your idea. Let your mind go; be creative with your ideas. Try summarizing the main idea of what you want to convey in your essay in one or two sentences or in those famous "25 words or less." These summary sentences will be useful in your introduction and/or conclusion. If you start early enough, you can take a few minutes a day for several days in this phase. And you can do it anywhere, such as while driving to work or washing the car. Just be sure that you jot down the ideas for later use.

During the brainstorming stage, jot down as many ideas as possible — you can never have too many ideas during brainstorming. In the outlining stage, however, you need to consider the length of the final paper. Almost all instructors specify length. Some instructors take off marks if a student writes a paper that is longer than specified. If at this point — *before* you begin to write — you consider the overall length, you can focus on the most important ideas and group the less important ideas so that you cover the greatest amount of information without putting too much emphasis on one point. You can decide to omit some details, or you can select one example to stand for several others. If you are conscious of length right from the beginning, likely you will not have to spend hours later trying to shorten a lengthy draft. As well, you will be less likely to ramble once you begin to write.

RUNG 4: CREATE (WORKING DRAFT)

If you spend time on the three early steps, then you should be able to write your first drafts for papers much more quickly than you have in the past. However, you should still plan on having to write out or type out at least one rough draft. Most professional writers say they need at least three.

This does not necessarily mean that you copy out your draft word-for-word each time. What you do is create a first "working copy" that you can go over several times. If you work on a computer, this is easy. You can alter your original draft quickly. However, even if you have not yet joined the computer generation, you can still create a working draft that is easy to alter. Write or type your first draft using only every second or third line (i.e., double- or triple-spaced), and use WIDE margins. (Many student nurses simply will not do this; they seem determined not to "waste" paper and thus cover every page from corner to corner, using every possible bit of space. Overcome this tendency!) If you double-space your writing, then you can go over the paper a second time (and third and fourth, if necessary) and simply add or delete words and phrases. You can write in the margins if you leave them wide enough. You can insert an asterisk (*) and turn the page over and add a sentence or two. You can cross out words and substitute better or clearer words above them. You can correct your spelling and grammar without having to crowd your words. You will be able to read your draft more easily and see if you have mistakes in grammar, spelling, or punctuation.

Ideally, you should create the first working copy quickly. A first draft should be creative and should flow. In early drafts, you concentrate on developing the main body of the message. From your brainstorming and outlining sessions, you know what the main points of your message are, and you will have organized them to make your message clear and strong, keeping your audience in mind. You should be able to pick up words and phrases directly from your brainstorming page and outline and incorporate them into the first draft.

You may still find it hard to start writing at this point. The best way is simply to begin. Put some sentences down on your paper or on the screen of your computer. Simply by writing half a page or more, you get started. You may eventually scrap it, but you have started. This approach is called "free writing."

During first-year nursing courses, some instructors give free writing or quick writing assignments in class. Students are asked simply to take a piece of paper and start writing down their thoughts. Such assignments help you to improve your writing and your thinking skills. These assignments are often described as "writing-to-learn" projects (as opposed to "learning-to-write" projects) and are designed to help student nurses acquire and interpret (for both themselves and others) the complex knowledge base that makes up nursing. For these projects, you still need to think SMART — but you do it quickly.

You can practise free writing or quick writing on your own. Writing things down helps you to clarify theoretical points or reflect on ways that personal experiences (sometimes called "lived experiences") can be applied. Such practice helps you to develop conceptual approaches and thinking patterns that will also be helpful in practice settings.

Once you are caught up in the flow of the writing, your thoughts will become more organized. Many writers like to complete the body of the paper first and then turn to the introduction and conclusion. Other writers like to write the introduction first because it helps them to clarify exactly what they want to say and the order in which to say it. Either way, you want to keep the introductory and concluding sections short, especially during the first draft. You can come back to them during the next steps when you edit and revise.

Writing the first draft is not the time to get out the dictionary and check spelling. If you do not know how to spell a word, simply draft it in and put (sp?) beside it so that you can check it later. Look quickly to see that you have the references on hand as you mention them in the draft, but do not worry about getting them copied down in detail; leave this for later.

At this point, you should be trying to put the message into your own words, showing that you truly understand what it is. Be creative, remembering that this is merely the *beginning* of the paper; knowing that this version does not have to be perfect helps you to let your ideas flow. Envision your instructor reading it. See it as a kind of long, informative letter with a specific message from you. Focus on getting your whole message across.

Once you have your first draft finished, try to leave it as is and take a break. If you can leave it overnight and do the editing and revising the next day, you will likely be able to read the paper over and easily spot areas that need to be worked on further. If you are organized enough to be preparing the paper several days in advance, then you will even have time to do a bit more research if necessary.

When you come back to your first draft, continue at first to concentrate on the message rather than on details of spelling and grammar. Ask yourself if you got the main point across clearly so that any reader could understand it. Are the subordinate points obvious so that the reader can follow them clearly? You may want to add more in one section, elaborate some point, or give an example to make your point clearly. If you work on a computer, these revisions are easy. If not, you can get the scissors and cut and paste or tape. All good writers have done this, from Charles Dickens to Ernest Hemingway.

Keep considering the length as you work. If you work on a computer, you will find it easy to work out the length. If you are still writing your papers by hand, count the number of words on a typical page and estimate the number of pages that you will need for the finished copy. Keep this number in mind for future papers. (If you must do a count, include all the little words such as "a," "the," and "I.")

Eventually, you will achieve a copy that contains the message you are satisfied with — or, more likely, you will run short of time! Either way, you need to go over the draft version once more.

RUNG 5: EDIT

During the final review of the draft, you stop creating the message and concentrate instead on critiquing and improving the writing. Now is the time to look at vocabulary, grammar, punctuation, and spelling. This is the time to consider the tone of the essay. Is it too formal? Have you used appropriate language for a college-level paper? Have you used the appropriate vocabulary for your level of nursing ("abdomen" rather than "tummy"; "intestine" rather than "gut")? Have you borrowed jargon from the readings without really understanding it? Are your words too pretentious? A general rule is that clear, simple, appropriate words convey your message the best. Use your critical faculties. Stop looking at what you want to say and concentrate on saying it well and clearly.

When you begin to revise, concentrate especially on good, clear writing in the introductory and concluding sections of the paper. They are vital because they make the most impact on readers. You want to start with some strong, clearly stated, and, if possible, memorable sentences. And you want to end your message by clearly reviewing what you tried to achieve in the body of the paper. The words of your final paragraph will leave a lasting impression on your instructor as he or she works out your mark. So consider these sections carefully. Many great authors suggest that you spend as much time on the first and the last paragraphs as you do on the rest of the paper!

A useful hint at this stage is to read the paper out loud to yourself, listening to the words and grammar rather than to the message. Does the sentence sound right, or can it be misinterpreted? Consider these newspaper headlines that slipped by editors:

"Miners Refuse to Work After Death"
"Drunken Drivers Paid $1,000 Last Week"
"Local High School Dropouts Cut in Half"

Watch out for sentences that are too long to read comfortably. Do you get lost halfway through a sentence? Do you fail to understand what a pronoun refers to? (If you have trouble with it, think how difficult it will be for your instructor or other readers!)

If the draft is not too messy, get someone else to read it — but either provide a photocopy or tell the person not to write on your version. (Give him or her some Post-it notes.) Try to find someone who is helpful but not overly critical; all writers are vulnerable when they give a draft to someone to review! The person need not be an expert on the content, but pick someone who can learn from reading your paper — and he or she will only learn from it if it is clearly written. You want a friend who will offer some praise and positive feedback as well as some useful critical comments. Remember, too, that you do not have to accept and use all the criticisms. Chapter 3 gives more detail on these and other points to look for when you are editing the final draft.

RUNG 6: SHINE (FINAL VERSION)

As you print out or type up the final copy — or just before you send it to the typist — look at the general format of the paper, such as headings, spacing, table of contents, size of type, and so on. Also consider your quotations, citations, and references. These are all points related to the route — and, for first-year student papers, they are covered in Chapters 4 and 5. If you are in a more senior year, you probably need a style manual that spells out the rules of the route in more detail. Or, if you are looking at the rules for other presentations (business letters, résumés, business reports), you may want to review Chapter 6.

You need to turn in a final version that is clean and easy to read. Just as you would not appear for a job interview in dirty, ragged gardening clothes, your paper must appear on the instructor's desk in a suitable form. Unless you have made other arrangements with the instructor, you should turn in a typed or printed paper. Some instructors will allow you to turn in a handwritten version, but it must also be clean. Even your handwritten version must follow the general rules for papers (i.e., double-spaced, with wide margins, on 8.5" by 11" white, unlined paper). If you type, be certain that you have a good typewriter or printer ribbon. This small investment is important, as I know from experience; if your paper is 59th in a pile of 75, the instructor's eyes will be tired and sore.

Some instructors like to receive assignments in folders or envelopes. If so, they will usually specify this in the assignment handouts. Sometimes the route specified in the assignment dictates what you use (e.g., you are to submit a nursing assessment on a Kardex or chart page). Most often, however, you should simply turn in an assignment paper as advised in the style sheet or manual recommended for use by your department. (Most style sheets and manuals suggest that you gather the pages together with a paper clip; a few recommend using a staple in the top left corner.) These rules are meant to make it easier for the instructor to carry, read, and mark up your assignment.

Instructors often want or need a few extra things in a student paper that may not be specified in a style manual. For example, a distance education student may decide to attach a cover letter (probably only a short note) to the paper. I have appreciated the cover letters that distance education students have included with papers sent to me. They allow you to give additional details that may not be appropriate in a formal paper. For example, the letter might explain why the paper is late (or early, as the case may be). Or you may need to indicate that you are going to be away temporarily and need to have the paper returned to some other address. If you use a cover letter, it should be set up properly as a business letter — although it need not be typed.

As a final step — providing you have time — you should read over the hard copy (the finished draft from the typist or from your computer printer) before you turn it in. You may find a few typing errors (e.g., "works" instead of "words") that slipped by previous proofreading. Or you may find a place where there was a small breakdown in the computer codes that caused minor errors or typos in a few words or lines. You can correct these mistakes neatly in ink on the final copy or use a clean eraser or a bit of "white out" solution to tidy up the page. You will not lose marks if you make the corrections clearly and neatly, but you probably will if you simply leave the typo or the error.

RUNG 7: SUBMIT (ON TIME)

The final step in the writing process is to submit the paper on time. Some instructors deduct marks for a paper that is late. One reason for doing so is that other students manage to meet the deadline, and if you do not you have an unfair advantage over them. On the other hand, most instructors will give you an extension when there is a real emergency, such as personal illness or a death in the family. Ask!

■ Summary

In this chapter, I have provided a number of ideas that are useful to writers, including some general hints and some information on using libraries. As well, I have described a specific writing process that has proven useful for a generation of student nurses. If you look back, you will see that the initial letters for each of the steps spell out PROCESS.

Plan
Research
Outline
Create
Edit
Shine
Submit

Remembering this acronym will help you to understand that good writing has several steps — and, if you want to write like a pro, the most important steps occur before you sit down to write. I have included self-assessment exercises on mapping and outlining to give you some practice using these two parts of the process.

● EXERCISE 2.1 *Brainstorming*

Try a five-minute brainstorming session and make a map of some topic for a 10-page college-level paper. You might try "My Favorite Flower," or "Making a Hospital Bed," or "Pros and Cons of Wearing a Uniform in Nursing," or any other topic.

● COMMENTS ON EXERCISE 2.1 *Brainstorming*

Refer to the map in Figure 2.2 for ideas about mapping. Following, however, are some points to keep in mind.

For each topic, you have some latitude — but even in this exercise you need to consider all the SMART elements. Let's say that the first "favorite flower" to spring to your mind is B.C.'s floral symbol, the flowering dogwood (*Cornus nuttallii*). If you are deeply interested in B.C. wildflowers and have an excellent personal library on them, developing such a topic for 10 pages would be relatively easy. However, if you have only a passing interest in flowers, you might have to do a great deal of research to write 10 pages. At this point, it might be wiser to decide to write about a rose; basic information about roses is easier to find, and you could devote some part of the paper to a discussion of the impact that roses have had on your senses (smell, texture) or on your life (you once gave a single red rose to a friend, who fell in love with you because of it!). Keep your audience in mind as well. Is this a paper for a botany class in which the instructor is likely extraordinarily knowledgeable about flowers and may question whether the dogwood tree should be classified as a flower? Or is it a paper for a psychology class in which your instructor would like to know about images and reactions?

● **EXERCISE 2.2** *Organization*

Look at Chapter 2 as if it were a student paper. Make an outline showing its organizational plan.

● **COMMENTS ON EXERCISE 2.2** *Organization*

The outline should look something like this:

I. Introduction
— general hints about and specific steps in the writing process; chapter will describe them and how they can aid in the preparation of student papers

II. Body
   A. General hints
      — a place for writing
      — tools
      — computers (a special tool)
      — avoiding procrastination

B. Using the library
  — books versus articles
  — computer catalogues and indexes
C. The writing process
  — describe the seven steps using acronym PROCESS

III. Summary
  — tell them what you told them
  — try to end with a memorable quote

■ References

Colombo, J. R. (Ed.). (1974). *Colombo's Canadian quotations*. Edmonton: Hurtig.

Dupuis, K. C., & Wilson, S. V. (1982). *Communicating with P.O.W.E.R.* Toronto: Gage.

Markman, R. H., Markman, P. T., & Waddell, M. L. (1994). *10 steps in writing the research paper* (5th ed.). Hauppauge, NY: Barron's Educational Series.

Common Errors
in Writing

Common errors are simple, everyday mistakes that you often find in the writings of non-professional writers — and even in the writings of some professional writers. You may hear some of these mistakes daily on your radio or read them in the popular press or magazines. You may even hear them in conversation with your instructors or in lectures. Think for a minute, however, about the SMART elements: usage is affected by route. The errors that I describe in this chapter are elementary ones that you should not make in formal college- or university-level papers. If you make these errors, they mark you as a careless, sloppy, "uneducated" writer.

Frequently, these common errors represent things that you can *say* (use appropriately, even in formal oral communications) but that are not appropriate in formal written communications. You may have heard the maxim "Write the way you talk"; that piece of good advice tells you to avoid seeming too pretentious. However, unless you speak as well as Winston Churchill did, you probably need to write slightly more formally in your papers. For example, you should avoid contractions (e.g., I'm, we've, can't, won't, shouldn't, it's) in college or university papers — unless you are quoting from another source or reproducing dialogue. So, when you are editing your paper, you need to look for these everyday errors.

In Chapter 2, I described the steps of the writing PROCESS, concentrating on the need for you to **P**lan, **R**esearch, and **O**rganize your information and on how you begin to **C**reate a first draft. I also briefly mentioned the steps of **E**diting, **S**hining up your prose, and **S**ubmitting your paper. In this chapter, I want to discuss in more detail those editorial and polishing steps — the ones you do after you have developed and drafted the content of your paper to your satisfaction. In learning to edit and shine your assignments, you need to look, in particular, at common errors made in written communications.

Although this chapter deals with some errors in grammar, this text is not intended to be a basic grammar book. As I mentioned in Chapter 1, if you have been accepted into a nursing-education program, you are expected to have good language, grammar, and writing skills. You should have, as reference tools, a good dictionary and one or two good basic grammar texts on your shelves to help you as you edit, revise, and polish your paper. Just how basic or how advanced your reference tools should be will depend on your present skills as a writer; choose the kind of book you need now, but be prepared to look for more advanced texts as you gain better writing skills through practice, reading, and feedback from your instructors. Appendix D gives notes on and recommends some useful reference books that might appeal to you.

You need to *fix* the following common errors before you type up the final version or send it to the typist. Allow yourself about an hour to go through the final draft, looking for

- long, complex sentences;
- passive (instead of active) voice;
- weak pronouns and verbs at start of sentences;
- long, complicated, or inappropriate words (jargon);
- lack of agreement of terms;
- lack of parallel structure;
- misused words;
- biassed language;
- unnecessary words; and
- inconsistencies in punctuation, spelling, and capitals.

■ Error: Long, Complex Sentences

A whole science of communications has grown up since the 1950s, and a great deal of research has been done into what Flesch (1960) has called "readability." Such research shows that people with high school and university educations are most comfortable reading sentences that average about 20 to 25 words. When a sentence contains 40 or more words, even people with doctoral degrees tend to get confused and disoriented, although if they are familiar with the subject matter, they can often follow the ideas. Clear words, logical flow, and good punctuation also help a reader to get through the maze. However, long sentences make readers tired and irritable. Do you want an irritable instructor marking your paper?

Reading your paper out loud often helps you to spot long sentences, although you can also find them simply by looking at the final draft. Usually, you can divide long sentences into two (or more) shorter sentences that convey your thoughts more clearly. You do not want to make all your sentences short; doing so will make your paper sound like a primary school assignment. Just take care that a sentence is not too long and that there are not many long sentences. Look critically at some of the articles you are required to read. When you need to reread passages because you seem to lose the meaning, you will usually find a long sentence as the culprit.

● EXERCISE 3.1 *Long Sentences*

Try reading the following long sentence, which actually appeared in a draft report written for the American Hospital Association.

> In addition to their primary mission of providing health care and related education to the sick and injured, hospitals have a responsibility to work with others in the community to assess the health status of the community, identify target health areas and population groups for hospital-based and cooperative health promotion programs, develop programs to help upgrade the health in those target areas, and ensure that persons who are apparently healthy have access to information about how to stay well and prevent disease, provide appropriate health education programs that aid those persons who choose to alter their personal health behaviour or develop a more healthful lifestyle, and establish the

hospital within the community as an institution which is concerned about good health as well as one concerned with treating illness.

Try rewriting the message. Refer to the following comments for suggestions.

● COMMENTS ON EXERCISE 3.1 *Long Sentences*

That sentence has 130 words in it. You could rewrite its message in several ways. The 122 words in the following version are divided into five sentences (two of which use semicolons, which help to turn the sentences into seven distinct thoughts); thus, this version is much easier to understand.

> In addition to a primary mission of providing care and related education to the sick and injured, hospitals have four goals. First, hospitals need to work with local individuals to assess the community's health status. Second, hospitals must help identify target health areas and population groups for hospital-based and co-operative health-promotion programs; they then develop programs to help upgrade health in those target areas. Third, hospitals also must ensure that apparently healthy persons have access to information about how to stay well and prevent disease; hospitals must provide appropriate health-education programs that aid people to alter their health behaviors and develop healthful lifestyles. Fourth, hospitals must be community institutions just as concerned with good health as with treating illness.

The following passage uses a different format to break up the message and make it easier for the reader to follow. It contains 128 words in two sentences, but the message is broken into seven distinct passages and is therefore easier to read.

> In addition to the primary mission of providing health care and related education to the sick and injured, hospitals have six other goals:
>
> - to work with others in the community to assess the health status of the community;
> - to identify target health areas and population groups for hospital-based and co-operative health-promotion programs;

- to develop programs to help upgrade health in those target areas;
- to ensure that persons who are apparently healthy have access to information about how to stay well and prevent disease;
- to provide appropriate health-education programs that aid those persons who choose to alter their personal health behavior or develop a more healthful lifestyle; and
- to be an institution within the community that is as concerned with good health as with treating illness.

■ Error: Passive Rather Than Active Voice

Use of active voice in writing gives strength and vitality to a sentence; passive voice slows things down. Passive voice is when the doer of the action in the sentence is not the subject of the main verb. Consider the following examples:

- A splendid coach was pulled by six black horses.
- The bed was pushed across the room.
- My first visit to Well Known Hospital will always be remembered.

Although communication research shows that passive voice is more confusing and tiring for readers, the first example is not a major problem for readers. The sentence is short and clear. Occasional use of such passive sentences is fine because they may give variety to your essay. The second example illustrates how passive voice creates problems that may be more serious. Ask yourself: "Pushed across the room by whom? Does the reader need to know this information?" In many instances, the reader does need to know such information; even if the reader does not need to know it, he or she might wonder who did the pushing and thereby become distracted from your real message. The last example illustrates the kind of problem that occurs when writers misuse the passive voice; the meaning of the sentence is not clear. Ask yourself "Remembered by whom?" The writer of that sentence probably meant "I will always remember my first visit to Well Known Hospital," although another meaning is certainly possible.

Some writers, including many researchers, tend to use (and misuse) passive voice in attempts to keep themselves in the background. In recent years, even researchers are advised to use first-person pronouns

(I or we) when necessary and to avoid passive voice. If they do not, they may get into difficulty with the meanings of sentences. In some of your nursing courses, such as charting (a different route than an essay or formal paper), you may be advised to "Keep yourself out of the report." However, you can still avoid passive voice and keep yourself in the background. Look at the following two sentences:

- Some statistics were found to be extraneous to the report but were put into the appendix. (Passive — found by whom? put by whom?)
- Some statistics did not apply to this report but are in the appendix. (Active)

The solution is to use active voice whenever you can. Watch for passive voice when you are checking your final drafts and change it when necessary.

Note that passive voice and past tense are different. A sentence in the active voice can be in the past tense. If you do not understand the difference, then refer to this point in a good basic grammar book. Try the following exercise.

● EXERCISE 3.2 *Passive Versus Active Voice*

In this exercise, sentences are in the passive voice; rewrite each one in the active voice.

1. A memo to head nurses, advising them of the workshop, was sent by the vice-president of nursing.

2. A copy of each prescription must be sent back to the ward with the drug from pharmacy.

3. The agenda for the meeting should be prepared by the representative from clinical pathology.

4. The purchasing department door was left unlocked by someone; this made it possible for the computer records to be picked up by mistake when the delivery man made his rounds.

5. Fire regulations must be explained to each new employee during the orientation week.

6. As he entered the hospital, the chairman of the board was hit on the head by a flowerpot falling from the window ledge above the door.

● COMMENTS ON EXERCISE 3.2 *Passive Versus Active Voice*

Most of these sentences could be rewritten in a number of ways, but the following show some of the easiest ways to repair each one. Think about each rewritten version. Is the active voice better in all revisions?

1. The vice-president of nursing sent a memo to head nurses, advising them of the workshop.
   OR
   The head nurses received a memo, advising them of the workshop, from the vice-president of nursing.
   In the original sentence, the main verb is part of *to send*. Ask yourself "Who sent the memo?" In the first rewrite, I put the doer of the sending in front of the verb. In the second rewrite, I changed the verb. The head nurses are now the doers of the verb *to receive*. Ask yourself "Who received the memo?"

2. Pharmacy staff must send a copy of each prescription back to the ward with the drug.

3. The representative from clinical pathology should prepare the agenda for the meeting.

4. Someone left the purchasing department door unlocked; this made it possible for the delivery man to pick up the computer records by mistake when he made his rounds.
   Note that I assisted you with this example because I put in the words *by someone*. But see what happens in the next example.

5. (Someone) must explain fire regulations to each new employee during orientation week.
   OR
   During orientation week, each new employee must attend a session with the hospital's fire marshall to learn the fire regulations.
   The original sentence was taken directly from Well Known Hospital's orientation manual. The problem at WKH, because passive voice is used in the original, was that no one was responsible for actually explaining the fire regulations! You cannot edit that sentence; you have to send it back to the writer and ask him or her to make it clear who is to do the explaining.

6. *A flowerpot, falling from the window ledge above the door, hit the chairman of the board on the head as he entered the hospital.* In this example, the flowerpot did the action, so this rewrite is in the active voice. However, the original sentence is probably better because it makes the content more relevant. So an additional warning is needed: do not become overly dependent on rules (even *my* rules!). Churchill was once told that he should not end a sentence with a preposition — and he replied: "That is the kind of nonsense up with which I shall not put." Think SMART.

■ Error: Weak Pronouns and Verbs

Poor writers tend to rely too often on pronouns (rather than nouns) and on weak beginnings to sentences. Such writing habits take all the vitality out of a written communication. For example, a pronoun often fails to convey the correct meaning.

> Students watched as instructors demonstrated the correct method for injecting medications into an intravenous tube. This is a common technique that they will be required to practise in the laboratory.

The pronoun *this* is intended to refer to the complete sense of the preceding sentence, but on first reading the pronoun seems to refer to "tube." Furthermore, the pronoun *they* later in the sentence can refer to either "students" or "instructors."

Sentences that begin with "This is ..." or "There are ..." — or with similar constructions (e.g., "These were ...," "There is ...," "That was ...") — are usually weak constructions and can be strengthened merely by editing. For example:

> There was a beautiful princess who lived at the edge of the forest.

This sentence would be better written as:

> A beautiful princess lived at the edge of the forest.

The solution is to use strong nouns and verbs. Watch for sentences beginning with the weak constructions and change them when possible. Many weak openings can simply be eliminated, as in the example above. Always watch for a pronoun (especially they, it, and this) at the beginning of a sentence, and be sure that the reference to the antecedent noun is clear. Try the following exercise.

● EXERCISE 3.3 *WEAK PRONOUNS AND VERBS*

Edit the following sentences.

1. There are two things that really bother me: weak pronouns and weak constructions.

2. Once upon a time, there were three little pigs who lived with their mother at the edge of the forest.

3. There are a variety of walkers which provide support to those who are weak and have difficulty maintaining balance. Some of these have wheels, although others need to be lifted with each step.

4. The nurses at Well Known Hospital use a variety of brochures, check lists, and instruction sheets to help patients learn postoperative techniques. They find the brochures are helpful and often use them to make notes about questions they need to discuss with their doctors.

● COMMENTS ON EXERCISE 3.3 *Weak Pronouns and Verbs*

Following are some ways to edit and improve these sentences.

1. Two things really bother me: weak pronouns and weak constructions.

2. Once upon a time, three little pigs lived with their mother at the edge of the forest.

3. A variety of walkers provide support to those who are weak and have difficulty maintaining balance. Some of the walkers have wheels, although others need to be lifted with each step.

4. The nurses at Well Known Hospital use a variety of brochures, check lists, and instruction sheets to help patients learn postoperative techniques. The patients find the brochures helpful and often use them to make notes about questions they need to discuss with their doctors.

Remember that this point is important in written communications. In oral presentations (a different route), good speakers often form a sentence with a weak beginning so that the emphasis comes at the end, when tone of voice can stress the point for listeners' ears. You probably remember that many fairy tales or children's stories prepared for reading aloud start with "Once upon a time, there was...."

■ Error: Long, Complicated, or Inappropriate Words

Short, clear, simple, direct words are better in your writing than long, complex ones that may confuse, tire, or hinder the reader. In informational writing, simple words have more impact than complex ones. Everyday words are easier for the reader to understand — and usually they are easier for the writer to spell correctly! Complex words are often jargon (also sometimes called gobbledegook, bafflegab, officialese, or newspeak). Jargon is a derogatory term; it applies when you write "utilize" for "use," or "debark," "deplane," or "off-load" instead of "leave" or "get off." Slang (e.g., dude), foreign terms (e.g., a priori, au courant), and out-dated words (e.g., whilst, amongst) can also be included in this category of inappropriate terms.

Note that jargon does not mean professional terms — unless, of course, they are not suited to your receivers. For example, "Are you suffering from an acute upper gastrointestinal tract inflammation?" is inappropriate when you want to ask a seven-year-old child "Do you have a tummy ache?" On the other hand, it would be entirely appropriate to write in the nurse's notes "The child shows symptoms of an acute upper GI inflammation." When you, a nurse, are writing for nursing colleagues or other health care professionals, you must use the appropriate words. However, it is wrong when you use words only to mystify or impress, or when you use terms to disorient or confound.

Often jargon reflects popular words used in the media and, especially, in advertising, but nursing has its jargon too. Examples include hospitalize, operationalize, bedrest patients, maximize, paradigms, therapeutic milieu, and conceptual frameworks. I am not saying that you should never use these words, but think SMART. Sometimes you (the source) may want to baffle or buffalo your readers (the audience). Some politicians frequently do this! Perhaps in some situations, you want to use big words to impress, but you must also consider the impact they may have on the reader. If an instructor gets the impression that you are using terms only to sound impressive, he or she may start looking into your sentences carefully for errors. Another problem is that misuse of words — and it is easy to misuse complicated terms — always fails to impress. When possible, stick to strong, clear, accurate, basic English. Try the following exercise.

● EXERCISE 3.4 *Long, Inappropriate Words*

Practise simplifying your language by giving shorter or easier equivalents for the words and phrases listed below.

utilize _____   achieve _____

attempt _____   ascertain _____

numerous _____   terminate _____

demonstrate _____   consult _____

purchase _____   reside _____

modification _____   explicit _____

subsequent _____   initial _____

accumulate _____   remainder_____

obliterate _____   indemnify_____

voluminous _____   endeavor _____

for the reason that _____ _____

her personal physician_____

he totally lacked the ability to _____

List three jargon terms or complex words that particularly bother you; then give their simpler equivalents.

1.
2.
3.

● COMMENTS ON EXERCISE 3.4 *Long, Inappropriate Words*

Following are some common substitutions. I originally compiled this list from words in quarterly reports filed by head nurses. Note the word *indemnify*. You should also check a dictionary for all the meanings before you substitute a word.

utilize	*use*
achieve	*get, gain*
attempt	*try*
ascertain	*make sure*
numerous	*many*
terminate	*end, fire*
demonstrate	*show*
consult	*ask*
purchase	*buy*
reside	*live*
modification	*change*
explicit	*clear*
subsequent	*next*
initial	*first*
accumulate	*gather, get*
remainder	*rest*
obliterate	*erase, rub out*
indemnify	*pay*
voluminous	*big, large, full*
endeavor	*try*
for the reason that	*because*
her personal physician	*her doctor*
he totally lacked the ability to	*he could not*

Some words that bother me are "impact" used as a verb (use "affect"); "hopefully," which is almost always misused (leave it out); and "irregardless" (there is no such word).

Note that you cannot always substitute. In the list above, "voluminous" does not *mean* the same thing as "big," "full," or "large"; in use, it gives the reader a sense that the noun described has many folds and a great volume of material. In a way, it implies all three of the shorter words. However, you are using jargon if you use "voluminous" to impress your reader or listener when "full" would do. Sometimes you deliberately try to impress your audience with big words. Such use is still jargon — but it may be acceptable in that instance. But such use does not usually work with instructors.

■ Error: Lack of Agreement of Terms

Lack of agreement of terms within a sentence most commonly occurs when the writer uses a singular noun and a plural verb (or vice versa), or a singular noun and a plural pronoun (or vice versa), or a singular pronoun followed by a plural pronoun (or vice versa). Whole chapters have been written on this problem in grammar textbooks. The APA (1994) *Manual* devotes several pages to examples of this common error.

Look at the sentences below, which should give you some idea of this problem.

- The data is collected by questionnaire. ("Data" is a plural noun, so you need to write "The data are collected....")
- The doctors always enters the hospital through the side door. (Plural noun subject with a singular verb.)
- The head nurse should take care to avoid sexist language in their quarterly reports. ("Nurse" is a singular noun; thus, the pronoun "their" should be singular ["his or her"], or the noun should be changed to a plural form.)

These three examples represent the most common problems with lack of agreement in sentences. Usually, these are simple errors that you make while concentrating on creating the content in the first (or second) draft. You start the sentence one way, then change your mind about the wording halfway through. Unfortunately, if you do not correct the sentence later, it will be grammatically incorrect. In the editing stage, you need to read your paper carefully to pick up such errors so that they do not get copied into the final version. These errors may also represent poor typing rather than poor grammar — but your audience does not know that. If you make too many such errors in assignments, your instructors will get a poor impression of your abilities. You may think that such errors do not occur often — but I find them in about 25% of all papers I edit (and not just from students).

Watch for these problems when you edit. Reading your paper aloud during the final draft — as if you were reading it to someone — often helps you to spot these errors. Try the following exercise.

● EXERCISE 3.5 *Lack of Agreement of Terms*

Correct the following sentences.

1. Everyone should bring a writing pad to their next class.

2. Marjorie and Mary, after spending the afternoon in classes, plans to spend the evening with their husbands.

3. The patient needs to sign a surgical consent form before the operation; if this criteria is not met, legal problems may arise.

4. For patients with HIV disorders, even a minor infection, such as sinusitis or flu, prove dangerous.

5. Spread of cancer cells by diffusion are prevalent in serous cavities such as the abdomen or pleura.

6. Careless disposal of needles and sharp instruments often result in injuries to hospital staff.

● COMMENTS ON EXERCISE 3.5 *Lack of Agreement of Terms*

There are various ways to correct the sentences. Here are some:

1. Every<u>one</u> (singular) should bring a writing pad to the next class.
   OR
   Every<u>one</u> should bring a writing pad to his or her next class.

2. Marjorie and Mary, after spending the afternoon in classes, <u>plan</u> to spend the evening with their husbands.

3. The patient needs to sign a surgical consent form before the operation; if this <u>criterion</u> is not met, legal problems may arise. (The word *criteria*, like *data*, is plural.)

4. For patients with HIV disorders, even a minor infection, such as sinusitis or flu, <u>proves</u> dangerous.
   OR
   For patients with HIV disorders, even minor <u>infections</u>, such as sinusitis or flu, prove dangerous.

5. Spread of cancer cells by diffusion <u>is</u> prevalent in serous cavities such as the abdomen or pleura.

6. Careless disposal of needles and sharp instruments often <u>results</u> in injuries to hospital staff.

■ Error: Lack of Parallel Structure

One of the most common errors in sentence structure is a failure to keep all elements that perform the same purpose within the sentence *in the same form* (i.e., *parallel*). This error is so common that grammar teachers have a little symbol — // — that they put in the margin to indicate faulty parallelism in a student paper.

Parallel structure allows readers to follow a list of items within the sentence clearly and quickly. Faulty parallel structure confuses and annoys the reader. For example, the following sentence indicates a lack of parallel structure.

Mary likes swimming, golfing, and to play tennis.

The sentence lists three things that are objects of the verb *likes* — but the three things are not given in the same grammatical form. The first two ("swimming," "golfing") are gerunds, but the last one ("to play") is an infinitive verb. To be correct, they should have the same (parallel) form. When they do not, the reader does a double-take and has to reread the sentence.

Correct: Mary likes swimming, golfing, and playing tennis.
Correct: Mary likes to swim, golf, and play tennis.
Correct: Mary likes to swim, to golf, and to play tennis.

Sometimes errors in parallel structure occur in the words you use to introduce a series of sentences, as in "First, ..." "Secondly, ..." "Third, ...";
to be parallel, these words should be "first, second, third" or "firstly, secondly, thirdly." Be alert to this problem when you are doing lists (as in job descriptions). Reading aloud also often highlights this problem.

The following two common (but simple) examples illustrate lack of parallel structure and the ways in which the sentences can be corrected.

Wrong: The lottery winner liked his new computer, his new car, and new swimming pool.
Correct: The lottery winner liked his new computer, his new car, and his new swimming pool.
Correct: The lottery winner liked his new computer, new car, and new swimming pool.
Correct: The lottery winner liked his new computer, car, and swimming pool.

Note that repetition of words may be helpful to the reader, and the first two correct examples may be easier to read than the last one. Repetition, whether explicit or implicit, provides a similarity of structure so that the reader knows what is happening.

Wrong: Mary was both required to give the intravenous drugs and to make the patient comfortable.
Correct: Mary was required both to give the intravenous drugs and to make the patient comfortable.

Correct: Mary was required to both give the intravenous drugs and make the patient comfortable.

Parallel structure sometimes requires you to understand and use common correlative constructions, such as "both ... and" or "not only ... but also" or "neither ... nor." As you will recall from your grade school days, these constructions are bound to one another.

Wrong: Frank was required not only to give the intravenous drugs but to make the patient comfortable.
Correct: Frank was required not only to give the intravenous drugs but also to make the patient comfortable.

Sometimes a sentence can get complex and require two sets of parallel structure, as in the following example.

Wrong: I will examine context of instruction, subject matter, resources, teacher and learner characteristics and objectives, then end with a brief summary.

The two main parts of the sentence ("I will examine ... then end ...") need the conjunction *and*. However, the list is also complex, so the reader can only guess its meaning. The following are possible correct constructions.

Correct: I will examine context of instruction, subject matter, resources, and teacher and learner characteristics and objectives, and then end with a brief summary.
Correct: I will examine context of instruction, subject matter, resources, teacher characteristics, learner characteristics, teacher objectives, and learner objectives, and then end with a brief summary.

Note that the "extra" comma before "and" in a series (which we discussed in Chapter 1) makes the list clearer.

The following is another example of the lack of parallel structure.

Wrong: The objectives of the course are to learn to: identify common mistakes in language; learn to set up a manuscript properly; accurately edit papers; and familiarity with spelling styles.

The punctuation here does not help.

Correct: The objectives of the course are to learn to identify common mistakes in language, set up a manuscript properly, edit papers accurately, and become familiar with spelling styles.

Exercise 3.6 gives a few more examples of problems with parallel structure. If they do not help you to understand parallel structure, then refer to a good grammar textbook.

● **EXERCISE 3.6** *Lack of Parallel Structure*

1. The nurse arranged a physical examination, advised the patient about better nutrition, and then she told him how to change the dressing.

2. You either should go to the doctor's office or go to the hospital's emergency room.

3. Wet bed linen should be changed immediately because dry linen helps to prevent skin irritation and promoting psychological well-being.

4. Nursing interventions for metabolic acidosis include recording of fluid intake and output; administration of alkaline solutions as ordered; sodium bicarbonate kept on hand for emergency use; and safety precautions if the patient is restless, confused, or convulsing.

5. The procedure for preparing hot packs, either by boiling or steaming, is similar to that for hot compresses.

● **COMMENTS ON EXERCISE 3.6** *Lack of Parallel Structure*

1. The nurse <u>arranged</u> a physical examination, <u>advised</u> the patient about better nutrition, and <u>told</u> him how to change the dressing.

2. You <u>either should</u> go to the doctor's office <u>or should</u> go to the hospital's emergency room.
OR
<u>Either go</u> to the doctor's office <u>or go</u> to the hospital's emergency room.
OR
You should go <u>either to</u> the doctor's office <u>or to</u> the hospital's emergency room.

3. Wet bed linen should be changed immediately because dry linen helps <u>to prevent</u> skin irritation and <u>to promote</u> psychological well-being.
OR
Wet bed linen should be changed immediately because dry linen helps <u>prevent</u> skin irritation and <u>promote</u> psychological well-being.

4. Nursing interventions for metabolic acidosis include <u>recording</u> of fluid intake and output; <u>administering</u> alkaline solutions as ordered; <u>having</u> sodium bicarbonate on hand for emergency use; and <u>implementing</u> safety precautions if the patient is restless, confused, or convulsing.

5. The procedure for preparing hot packs, <u>either by</u> boiling <u>or by</u> steaming, is similar to that for hot compresses.
   OR
   The procedure for preparing hot packs, by <u>either</u> boiling <u>or</u> steaming, is similar to that for hot compresses.

■ Error: Misused Words

Good writers generally have good vocabularies. They know a large number of words and select the most accurate one to convey meaning clearly and succinctly. For example, a good writer would know (or look up in a dictionary) the difference between a dock, a pier, and a wharf. The primary meaning for "dock" is the area of water next to a wharf or pier; a "pier" is a structure that projects out into the water from the shore; a "wharf" is a platform built along the shore (i.e., parallel to the shore). You can take a walk along a wharf, but beware if someone advises you to "Take a long walk on a short pier" or to "Go walk on a dock."

As well, good writers have learned to distinguish between homonyms (words that sound the same but have different meanings), such as "rose" (past tense of the verb *rise*) and "rose" (the flower), or "hanger" (on which you hang clothes) and "hangar" (in which you put a plane). You are expected to have learned these differences before you were admitted to a nursing program. However, almost every writer has some problems; once you know what they are, you can resolve them or avoid them. Here are the 10 that I find frequently in nursing students' papers — with some advice on fixing them during the editing and polishing stages.

IT'S VERSUS ITS

Many writers (I am shocked at the number) have a problem with *its* and *it's*. The following is correct: "Nursing has its problems, but usually it's wonderful to care for patients." The word *its* is a possessive pronoun; the word *it's* is a contraction of "it is" (or, occasionally, of "it has"). Many students complain that it seems odd (or illogical) that the possessive pronoun does not take an apostrophe, as in "nursing's problems," "boy's book," or "John's dog." However, in "his book" or "the dog is hers," there are no apostrophes. You need to think of the possessive pronoun *its* as being like "his" or "hers."

You can also use another rule. You should avoid contractions in formal writing (you can also avoid many of them in informal writing without any problem). Therefore, if you are polishing your paper, check each time you have *its* or *it's*. If you can substitute "it is" or "it has," make the substitution and avoid the contraction. If you cannot substitute "it is" (or "it has"), use *its* (with no apostrophe). In other words, the word *it's* (with the apostrophe) would never appear in your paper! Of course, if the contraction is within a quotation from another source, you need to leave it; just be certain that you have copied it correctly.

Please note that there is no such word as *its'*.

WHICH VERSUS *THAT*

An old joke says "Editors so often substitute *that* for *which* that they should be referred to as 'which-hunters.'" The two words have different meanings; both are pronouns, but *that* is restrictive or defining, and *which* is non-restrictive or non-defining. In conversations (one route), *which* is frequently substituted for *that*, but the meaning is made clear from the way in which the speaker pauses (or fails to pause) within the sentence or from inflections in the voice. In written communications (another route), the words themselves, aided by punctuation, must convey the meaning. So, because the two words have different meanings, good writers need to know when to use *which* and when to use *that*. Consider these examples:

- The pharmacy, which is on the first floor, is closed on Sunday.
- The pharmacy which is on the first floor is closed on Sunday.
- The pharmacy that is on the first floor is closed on Sunday.

The first sentence says that there is only one pharmacy in the hospital and that it is closed on Sunday. In the second example, the meaning is not clear, but without the commas most editors would assume *which* should be *that* and make the substitution. The third sentence implies that there may be more than one pharmacy, but the restrictive clause adds defining information; it means that the one on the first floor is closed on Sunday.

The third example can be rewritten in a way that would make the sentence shorter but just as clear:

The first-floor pharmacy is closed on Sunday.

One good way to determine when you should use *which* is to read the sentence and see if it makes sense if you omit the non-restrictive *which*-clause. If the sentence makes sense without the clause, then use *which*, but be sure to add commas around the clause to make it completely clear to your readers. If you cannot omit the clause, then change the *which* to *that*. In other words, be your own which-hunter.

WHILE

Many students use the word *while* incorrectly when they really should use *although* or *but* or *whereas*. The error is simple to correct. The noun *while* means "time" (as in "for a *while*"). When *while* is used as a subordinating conjunction (i.e., when it ties another clause into the sentence), it still has a connotation of "time" and usually means "at the same time as." The old saying "Nero fiddled while Rome burned" is accepted as correct; "Nero fiddled while I played the piano" is only correct if I know another Nero and we are doing a duet! A good writer therefore uses *while* only when it has a timely meaning. Note the differences in meaning in the following examples.

- While I gave the medications, the doctor wrote the orders.
- Although I gave the medications, the doctor wrote the orders.
- The doctor wrote the orders while I gave the medications.
- The doctor wrote the orders, but I gave the medications.
- The doctor wrote the orders, whereas I gave the medications.

It is worth your while to learn the distinctions between *while* and *although*, *whereas*, and *but*.

DUE TO (WHEN IT SHOULD BE BECAUSE OF)

The word *due* is an adjective, not a conjunction, and the sentence must contain a noun to which *due* applies. Misuse of the phrase *due to* bothers many readers, although its use in conversation and informal writing is becoming more acceptable. Can you appreciate the differences below?

Correct: The cheque is due to arrive in the mail.
Correct: Her late arrival was due to the snowy weather. (But this sentence is clumsy and could be rewritten!)
Wrong: Due to the snow, she was late.

If you do not understand why the first two are correct, you need to watch for this phrase when you are editing your final drafts. Look carefully at the sentence in which the phrase is used; if you can substitute *because of* for *due to*, then do so!

FEEL (WHEN YOU MEAN *BELIEVE*)

In most dictionaries, the primary definitions for the word *feel* relate to "touch" rather than to "sense" or "consider." Good writers thus tend to restrict the use of *feel* to the primary meanings.

Correct: Feel the texture of his skin.
Correct: She feels her way across the darkened room.
Wrong: I feel this woman is ready to go to the delivery room.
Correct: I believe (or think) this woman is ready to go to the delivery room.

MAJORITY

This word is also commonly misused in conversation and in many news stories; students tend to use it unthinkingly in formal assignments. *Majority* means the larger (of two) and thus means "more than half" or "50% plus one" or "the greater part." You cannot have "a 40% majority"; in this instance, the word should be "plurality" (or you could say "won with 40% of the votes"). The same distinctions apply to the word *most* in good writing; be sure that you mean "more than half" when you use it. Also weigh the use of *many* (as in "Many patients ..."). Try to be specific when you use these words.

BETWEEN VERSUS AMONG

Back in grade school, you were taught the difference between these two words. *Between* relates to *two* people or things; *among* relates to *more than two*. You and I might keep a secret between us — but, according to the old adage, if we each tell another person, it becomes more difficult to keep something secret among three or more!

AFFECT VERSUS EFFECT

Affect is the verb; *effect* is the noun.

Correct: Does a high pollen count *affect* you? What *effect* does it have?

Simply knowing that these terms commonly create problems allows you to check their use. If you have a problem with them, then avoid using them by substituting other words. I have a problem knowing whether I should use *choose* or *chose*, so I frequently substitute the word *select*.

TO, *TOO*, AND *TWO*

I have never had a problem with these three homonyms, but studies show that they are among the three most common problems in business writing in the 1990s (along with *it's* versus *its*). If these words are problems for you, then consult a good dictionary until you finally achieve an understanding of them.

THERE VERSUS *THEIR*

The third most common error in business writing is the interchange of these two pronouns. The word *their* is a personal pronoun from the same family as *they*; *there* is similar to *this* or *that*. Consult a good grammar book if you have problems with this pair.

Exercise 3.7 illustrates a few more of these problems and gives you a chance to assess your vocabulary.

● EXERCISE 3.7 *Misused Words*

Choose the right word in each of the following options.

1. The administrator said it was a matter of (principal, principle) with her to pay only the (principal, principle) on the loan and not the interest.

2. Joan and Mary (alternately, alternatively) checked Mrs. Green's intravenous line and monitored Mr. Smith's blood pressure and pulse.

3. Tim thought it more (discreet, discrete) to wait until he was asked for help rather than (flaunt, flout) his superior strength.

4. The drug had some (adverse, averse) side-effects, causing the patient to break out in a rash.

5. Rani (lead, led) the way down the corridor.

6. She gave the report to Grace and (I, me, myself).

7. She expects to be promoted (some time, sometime) soon.

● **COMMENTS ON EXERCISE 3.7** *Misused Words*

The sentences should read as follows.

1. The administrator said it was a matter of principle with her to pay only the principal on the loan and not the interest.
   (*Principle* means "a rule of conduct" or "a basic truth"; *principal* in this usage means "the amount borrowed, as opposed to the interest on it," but can also mean "most important, main," and "head of a school.")

2. Joan and Mary alternately checked Mrs. Green's intravenous line and monitored Mr. Smith's blood pressure and pulse.
   (*Alternately* means "by turns"; *alternatively* means "choice" — and it might be simpler and clearer to say "Joan and Mary took turns checking Mrs. Green's intravenous line and monitoring Mr. Smith's blood pressure.")

3. Tim thought it more discreet to wait until he was asked for help rather than flaunt his superior strength.
   (*Discreet* means "tactful or prudent" and implies using good judgment in conduct; *discrete* means "separate or distinct"; *flaunt* means "to display blatantly, to show off"; *flout* means "to show contempt or scorn.")

4. The drug had some adverse side-effects, causing the patient to break out in a rash. (*Adverse* means "harmful or unfavorable"; *averse* means "opposed or reluctant.")

5. Rani led the way down the corridor. (*Lead*, pronounced to rhyme with "bead," is the present tense of the verb *to lead* and is only pronounced to rhyme with "red" when it is used as a noun to indicate the chemical substance.)

6. She gave the report to Grace and me.

7. Either is correct, although *sometime* (an adverb meaning "at an indefinite point of time") is more common in Canada.

■ Error: Biassed Language

In recent years, good writers have had to be conscious of using biassed language. Such language represents stereotypes that unintentionally creep into writing and that may offend or even insult readers.

Common biasses usually represent sexist language or deal with cultural, religious, or racial terms. As well, nurses and nursing students need to be aware of biasses in terms used to describe disabilities or health-related categories.

Nursing students in particular need to be aware that avoiding biassed language is more than just being politically correct; good use of language can promote social well-being and help you and others to have better self-esteem. If you refer to a patient with diabetes as "a diabetic" or to a child with epilepsy as "an epileptic," you can sound as if you are using a judgmental label. If you practise avoiding biassed terms in your writing, then you will also be more aware of them in oral communication.

Perhaps because 97% of nurses (and about 80% of nursing students) are female, female nursing students tend to make more mistakes with sexist language than other university students. Such habits are hard to break. Most female nurses tend to write "The nursing student must be aware of the needs of all her patients." The usually accepted alternatives for the sentence above are "The nursing student must be aware of the needs of all of his or her patients" and "Nursing students must be aware of the needs of all their patients."

Sexist language, like other forms of sexism, hurts, and nurses, simply because most of them are female and should understand the stigma of sexism, should avoid using sexist language.

Furthermore, colleges and universities have taken strong stands against sexist language and have advised all faculty members to be alert to this problem. Your instructors will likely notice, comment, and maybe take off marks if you refer to nurses exclusively as females.

Whole books have been written on sexist language and how to avoid it, such as *The Handbook of Nonsexist Writing*, by Miller and Swift (1988). Style manuals usually contain a section devoted to sexist language. The *Publication Manual of the American Psychological Association* (APA, 1994), for example, has several pages on this (as part of a larger problem of "bias") and an excellent table that gives some suggestions on how to avoid it. If you do not own an APA *Manual*, locate one in the library and read this section.

A common way to avoid sexist phrasing is to make your nouns plural. Thus, you would write "Nurses are concerned about their work environments" rather than "The nurse is concerned about his or her work environment." Use of the plural also helps you to avoid what I call the "everynurse syndrome" of writing, as if there were just one supernurse involved.

The following exercise gives you some practice in noticing, editing, and avoiding biassed language. Being aware of this problem will help you to avoid it.

● **EXERCISE 3.8** *Biassed Language*

Part A

The sentences below use biassed terms. Try editing or rewriting them to avoid sexist terminology.

1. The head nurse should ensure that her nursing staff attend CPR drills once a year.

2. When an anesthetist makes his rounds the evening before surgery, he needs to check with the evening admitting clerk to see if she has the list for the day surgery.

3. Every student at the University of Victoria has his name entered in the main computer.

4. To be admitted to the unit, a handicapped child must be able to dress and feed himself.

5. Dr. Alice Baumgart, past president of CNA, has been named chairman of the HEAL Committee.

6. When the new wing opens, the manpower needs of the hospital will increase 10%.

7. The telephone repairman removed the manhole cover so that he had easier access to the lines.

8. The man and his wife were upset when they found the flat tire.

Part B

Following are some common words that are suitable if you are referring to one individual and the sex is known, but that are sexist when the individual is not known. Try to supply a term that would be an acceptable non-sexist alternative.

waiter, waitress   _____

alderman   _____

spokesman, spokeswoman _____

steward, stewardess   _____

mailman   _____

weatherman, weather girl _____

fireman   _____

poet, poetess   _____

● COMMENTS ON EXERCISE 3.8 *Biassed Language*

There are several ways that you can fix the sexist writing. The following examples should help you to begin thinking about the appropriate use of words.

1. The head nurse should ensure that the nursing staff attend CPR drills once a year. (OR Head nurses should ensure that their nursing staff....)

2. When the anesthetist makes rounds the evening before surgery, he or she needs to check with the evening admitting clerk to see if the day surgery list is ready.

3. Every student at the University of Victoria has his or her name entered in the main computer. (OR Students at the University of Victoria have their names....)

4. To be admitted to the unit, a child with a handicap must be able to eat and get dressed without help. **(This version avoids the tiresome "himself or herself.")**

5. Dr. Alice Baumgart, past president of CNA, has been named chair of the HEAL Committee. (OR ... named to chair the HEAL Committee.)

6. When the new wing opens, the workforce needs of the hospital will increase 10%. (OR ... the personnel needs....)

7. The telephone repairer removed the utility-hole cover so that access to the lines was easier.

8. The husband and wife were upset when they found the flat tire. (OR The man and woman were upset....) **Some readers find the phrase "man and his wife" offensive because it suggests that the woman is defined in a possessive relationship. The parallel structure of "man and woman" or "husband and wife" is preferred.**

Part B

Following are some acceptable non-sexist alternatives.

waiter, waitress	*server, waiter* (waiter is often recommended for both)
alderman	*councillor* (councillor has been officially adopted by many city and municipal councils)
spokesman, spokeswoman	*representative* ("spokesperson" may be acceptable depending on your audience)
steward, stewardess	*flight attendant* (for unions, steward is used for both sexes; steward is also used for both sexes on ships)
mailman	*mail carrier*
weatherman, weather girl	*weather forecaster*
fireman	*fire fighter* ("stoker" is used for trains and ships)
poet, poetess	*poet* (poet is recommended for both sexes)

These are terms discussed fully in *The Handbook of Nonsexist Writing*, by Miller and Swift (1988). I recommend this book as solid reading when you have time. If you do not have time, then be aware that sexist terminology is not acceptable at the college level.

■ Error: Unnecessary Words

You should always edit out unnecessary words, leaving sentences tighter, crisper, clearer, and easier to read. In your first draft, you may write a sentence such as the following:

> An example of this problem is the fact that fever patients need increased rest and increased fluid intake.

During editing, you could rewrite the sentence as follows:

> For example, fever patients need increased rest and increased fluids.

Most grammar books contain long lists of wordy phrases. The following are just a few examples of phrases that could be pared down.

- in order to (just plain *to* usually does the job)
- at the present time (use *now* if anything)
- at this point in time (use *now*)
- the reason why (*the reason*)
- for the reason that (*because, since*)
- in the event that (*if*)
- are of the opinion that (*believe*)
- consensus of opinion (*consensus*)

Please watch for "in order to"; if you cannot substitute *to*, then the sentence may have a more serious problem!

Speakers (especially politicians responding to questions) tend to use long, unnecessary opening phrases to give themselves time to get their thoughts in order. Writers can organize their thoughts before they write, then edit so that readers can gain the essential message more easily. Watch for these phrases:

- It goes without saying that ... (then do not say it!)
- It is interesting to note that ... (is the rest of your paper not interesting?)

The word *the* is a special example. Many writers tend to overuse *the*. Obviously, sometimes you need to use *the* or your sentence will be unclear or ungrammatical. Do read over your sentences, however, and see if you can remove this little word. Look at the following examples:

- The staff at the Smithview Hospital set up additional beds in the hallways when the ambulances began arriving with the victims from the air crash.
- Staff at Smithview Hospital set up additional beds in hallways when ambulances began arriving with victims from the air crash.

In the second version, four of five *the's* were removed. The sentence still makes the same point, but it is much easier to read. When shining up your final drafts, look carefully for such extra words and cross them out. After a couple of years of practice, you will not even put them in!

Clichés are worn-out phrases that have been used too often. Originally, these phrases created images that sparked a reader's imagination. When they become commonplace, they no longer do that, and you need to weigh their use carefully. Either come up with a more exciting descriptive phrase that will make your paper memorable or leave out the cliché entirely. Some of the more common clichés I have found in student papers recently include the following.

- the bottom line
- quick as lightning
- good as gold
- the whole can of worms
- pretty as a picture
- quiet as a church mouse

Clichés indicate that you are a lazy writer. Avoid worn-out phrases, and be original in your expressions.

You should also avoid lazy words that creep into your writing but that fail to make any impact on the reader. In my writing workshops, I used to have all participants stand up, place the left hand over the heart, raise the right hand, and take the following pledge:

> I solemnly swear
> that I shall never use,
> in my writing,
> that terrible, four-letter word
>
> *very.*

Participants had a lot of trouble with that final word; they could not understand why I was making such a big point over *very*. However, even years later, I have had nurses come up to me to say that they have become better writers because they took that pledge and that they still feel guilty whenever they are tempted to write *very*. I know this seems simplistic, but if you, too, follow this rule, your writing will improve.

If you take the pledge to give up *very*, you will be forced to think about your vocabulary. And that means you will take a big step on the road to improvement in your writing.

Very is the worst of a long list of lazy words that weaken your writing. Others include *quite, rather, some, lots, many,* and *few*. Think about these words for a minute. How much smaller than small is very small or rather small? If you mean tiny, minute, microscopic, or infinitesimal, then use one of those words — or, in writing, just use small on its own. Is very big as accurate as gigantic, enormous, huge, 298 pounds, six foot seven inches, or 32 billion? When you are speaking, you can use body language (e.g., raise your eyebrows) and tones of voice (e.g., drawl the word *very*) to convey meaning. In your writing, however, *very* just signals that the following word was not strong enough on its own. Substituting the word *extremely* is no better either; you have just used a bigger word to get around the real problem.

Think, as well, about misuse of *very*. If you write, "She was a very honest nurse," does that imply there are degrees of honesty?

The correct solution is to use strong, accurate, descriptive nouns, adjectives, and verbs. When you go over your paper during the editing or polishing phase, look for lazy words. Try the following exercise.

● EXERCISE 3.9 *Unnecessary Words*

Look over the following sentences and simply cross out lazy words that add nothing to the paragraph.

1. Nurses very often neglect to mention quite obvious hazards when they are teaching patients to walk with a cane.

2. The implementation of these findings has been slow.

3. In order to write well, remove all extraneous and superfluous words.

4. The day was extremely frigid. Rather than spend quite a long time dressing all the residents in their outdoor clothes to take them out for some exercise, the nursing staff decided to hold a dance in the recreation room.

● COMMENTS ON EXERCISE 3.9 *Unnecessary Words*

This exercise was set up to help you find unnecessary words; almost all the sentences could be rewritten to make them stronger.

1. Nurses ~~very~~ often neglect to mention ~~quite~~ obvious hazards when they are teaching patients to walk with a cane.

2. ~~The~~ implementation of these findings has been slow.

3. ~~In order~~ to write well, remove ~~all extraneous and~~ superfluous words.

4. The day was ~~extremely~~ frigid. Rather than spend ~~quite~~ a long time dressing ~~all the~~ residents in ~~their~~ outdoor clothes to take them out for ~~some~~ exercise, ~~the~~ nursing staff decided to hold a dance in the recreation room.

■ Error: Inconsistencies in Punctuation, Spelling, and Capitalization

During the editing and polishing phases, you should review punctuation, spelling, and capitalization. You should look especially for inconsistencies.

Problems related to inconsistencies in spelling style were discussed in Chapter 1, and this final review is a good time to recall them. While creating the message, you may read several books and journals. If so, you may carry the style used in your readings into your paraphrases, writing "a woman in labor" on one page and "the labour and delivery room" a few pages later. Note that *judgement* (with an *e*) and *judgment* are both correct. Which is the more common in Canada? In the United States? In Britain? Which is recommended in the dictionary you use? The APA *Manual* recommends that you follow the spelling used in *Webster's* dictionaries, but many Canadian colleges and universities recommend that the *Gage* dictionaries be used as spelling guides. Usually, your instructors are not dogmatic about spelling style as long as you are consistent throughout the paper.

You also need to watch the style used in punctuation, another problem area mentioned in Chapter 1. You have to decide — based on Source * Message * Audience * Route * Tone — which punctuation style to use. For example, you need to decide whether to use a comma before the *and* in a series of three or more items — as in "We bought apples, oranges(,) and bananas." This is a matter of style, but in formal academic writing the comma usually goes in before *and*. In many journals and most newspapers, this comma is omitted. The APA *Manual* recommends the use of this comma; if you are going to use APA style, then watch for this point. You must be consistent in the way you use the comma.

In North America, the period (and most other punctuation marks) go inside the quotation marks — unless the meaning would be altered. As you create a rough draft, however, do not worry about the position of a period. As you do the critical review in the editing and polishing stages, you should look at the position of every punctuation mark.

Use of hyphens is partly a style matter and partly a spelling matter. Would you write "Nurses are concerned about a patient's *well-being*" (or use *wellbeing* or *well being*)? Think about the following alternatives.

- caregiver OR care-giver
- lifestyle OR life-style
- president elect OR president-elect
- postoperative or post-operative

Compound words take many styles: some are written as two words; some are joined as one word; some are hyphenated. Furthermore, some vary depending on their usage in the sentence (e.g., "The lab did an occult-blood test" but "The lab tested for occult blood"). The best tool to help you with hyphens is a good dictionary. You should decide which dictionary to use and look up the word. Remember, however, that when phrases are used in different ways, the spelling or hyphenation may change.

- Public health nurses give follow-up care.
- Public health nurses follow up clients.
- Instructors often use role playing in their classes.
- Role-playing techniques offer students opportunities to learn in non-stressful (nonstressful) situations.

Most style manuals recommend using hyphenated phrases only when necessary for clarity. The usual problem is that students are not consistent and sometimes use a hyphen, then later do not use a hyphen in the same word used the same way in a sentence. Watch — and be consistent!

Another area in which students are frequently inconsistent concerns capital letters. Some of the problems in determining when to use capital letters were mentioned in Chapter 1. You will face a number of decisions every time you write. For example, if you are writing a paper outlining recent changes in the organization of the Canadian Nurses Association, you might write something like the following:

At the Annual Meeting of the Canadian Nurses Association in June, the Board of Directors voted to replace the Advisory Council formerly representing its 22 Interest Groups with a new National Nursing Forum. The board decided that the forum would allow interest groups to speak with a united voice on matters and allow better communication among the groups on issues such as Liability Insurance.

At the annual meeting of the Canadian Nurses Association in June, the board of directors voted to replace the advisory council of its 22 interest groups with a new national nursing forum. The Board decided that the Forum would allow Interest Groups to speak with a united voice on matters and allow better communication among the groups on issues such as liability insurance.

In both the above passages, there are inconsistencies. Either style — one using an "up style" with capital letters and the other using a "down style" — is correct, depending on the decision of the writer. However, once that decision is made in the first sentence, the second sentence should be consistent with the determined style. Either of the following would then be correct:

> At the Annual Meeting of the Canadian Nurses Association in June, the Board of Directors voted to replace the Advisory Council formerly representing its 22 Interest Groups with a new National Nursing Forum. The Board decided that the Forum would allow Interest Groups to speak with a united voice on matters and allow better communication among the Groups on issues such as Liability Insurance.

> At the annual meeting of the Canadian Nurses Association in June, the board of directors voted to replace the advisory council of its 22 interest groups with a new national nursing forum. The board decided that the forum would allow interest groups to speak with a united voice on matters and allow better communication among the groups on issues such as liability insurance.

Usually, the decision is a matter of style. The most important point is that you need to be consistent in style throughout your paper. If you decide to use capital letters, then use them consistently. But should this decision about style be yours? As noted in Chapter 1, style can be affected by Source * Message * Audience * Route * Tone. In making decisions about style for formal student assignments, two important elements of The SMART Way need to be considered: audience and route. Has your instructor told you either in class or in the course syllabus that you are required to use a certain style manual (e.g., the APA *Manual* or some other manual or style sheet recommended by your college or university as a guide for student papers)? If so, then you should use it.

Even if your instructor has not specified a style manual, the route itself may dictate that you use one. When you were in high school, your assignments required a certain form, but that form is not what is required at college or university. The level of papers rises, and you are probably not well enough versed on the style decisions required. Style for college-level papers involves many elements! Even if your nursing program does not require you to use one style manual, I still suggest that you purchase one and learn how to use it. If you can make your own choice, then I recommend the APA *Manual*. It will be useful in many ways. For example, one of the most important concerns with college and university nursing papers is how to treat references. In

Chapter 4, I will go over the most important of these concerns and give you the basics of style for the first levels of college assignments, but a style manual is still a useful tool to own.

Exercise 3.10 gives you an opportunity to catch some inconsistencies in hyphenation. Try it.

● **EXERCISE 3.10** *Inconsistencies in Punctuation, Spelling, and Capitalization*

The following two paragraphs contain many common compound words or phrases. The paragraphs contain some repetition and some informal words, and they certainly could be edited to make the sentences stronger. However, the exercise should get you thinking about rules for hyphens. Simply insert hyphens where necessary.

> The vicepresident (nursing) decided that it was time to upgrade her 10 year old, workworn computer system by adding an up to date hard drive with a builtin modem. She called a face to face meeting with the hospital's computer programmer and the secretary from the human relations department. She preferred meetings rather than writing one page memos or using email; as well, with a meeting she could obtain feedback.
>
> As her staff arrived for the meeting, she thought how lucky she was to have such a hardworking group (not a donothing or clockwatcher among them). She said that her aboutface on computer replacement came when the old fashioned software system she had been using let two hyphens slip by her Xray vision. She said that she felt a loss of self esteem, and it was all downhill for the old fashioned system after that.

● **COMMENTS ON EXERCISE 3.10** *Inconsistencies in Punctuation, Spelling, and Capitalization*

I used hyphens based on the use recommended in *Gage Canadian Dictionary* (de Wolf, Gregg, Harris, & Scargill, 1997). Other dictionaries or style manuals may recommend other usage.

> *The vice-president (nursing) decided that it was time to upgrade her 10-year-old, workworn computer system by adding an up-to-date hard drive with a built-in modem. She*

called a face-to-face meeting with the hospital's computer pro-
grammer and the secretary from the human relations department. She preferred meetings rather than writing one-page
memos or using e-mail; as well, with a meeting she could
obtain feedback.

As her staff arrived, she thought how lucky she was to have
such a hardworking group (not a do-nothing or clockwatcher
among them). She said that her about-face on computer
replacement came when the old-fashioned software system
she had been using let two hyphens slip by her X-ray vision.
She said that she felt a loss of self-esteem, and it was all
downhill for the old-fashioned system after that.

■ Summary

The final review of your draft is an important step. Usually, you need
all your major writing tools (dictionary, style manual, grammar book)
at hand for this review. And it can take some time, which means that
you need to plan your assignments so that you allow time for this
step.

Fortunately, you will get much faster with practice, and what are
now definite, separate, time-consuming steps will soon become second
nature. For example, you should soon stop writing "very" and start
thinking about the most accurate word even as you write the first draft.
You will be alert to parallel structure when you start to make a list. You
will be envisioning your readers while you are drafting and therefore
starting to make your language suitable to your audience.

You may think that all this sounds like nit-picking. Remember, however, what nits really are. If you do not pick them out, you end up with
a lousy paper!

■ References

American Psychological Association. (1994). *Publication manual of the
American Psychological Association* (4th ed.). Washington, DC:
Author.

de Wolf, G. D., Gregg, R. J., Harris, B. P., & Scargill, M. H. (1997). *Gage
Canadian dictionary* (rev.). Toronto: Gage.

Flesch, R. (1960). *How to write, speak, and think more effectively.* New York: New American Library.

Miller, C., & Swift, K. (1988). *The handbook of nonsexist writing* (2nd ed.). New York: Harper & Row.

References and Bibliographies

If you (source) are not an expert in a subject, you may need to substantiate information presented to the reader (audience), especially if the information (message) is controversial, theoretical, or new. Usually, you take information from a reliable source, such as a research report or an expert, and include it to support your views. To do this properly in a formal paper (route), you need to understand the use of references and bibliographies.

References and bibliographies are essential components of college- and university-level papers. Furthermore, the need for good references and bibliographies increases throughout your nursing program. In your first-year papers, you may use only a few references, but you will use more in second-year papers. If you are in a baccalaureate course, your use of references will increase markedly in your third- and fourth-year courses. Furthermore, on graduation, when you use evidence-based nursing in your work, you may need to use references on the job. If you decide to take a master's degree, you will need to be familiar with several styles of references and bibliographies.

This chapter is intended to give you a sound introduction to references and bibliographies and to introduce you further to the mysteries of style manuals. The brief summary here will suffice for most first-year papers, but you also need to consider buying a good style manual as a reference tool.

In this chapter, I describe areas where nursing students just starting their programs often have difficulties with references. This information will likely suffice for all the papers you do during the first year, although eventually you should learn how to use a good style manual. This chapter also provides basic background information that usually is not included in style manuals. In particular, I describe briefly why a reference is used, introduce both the author-year and the numerical methods of citing references, explain what a complete citation includes, and outline the differences between reference lists and bibliographies. As well, I deal with the special instance of personal communications, which relate to information that you receive person to person, such as in an interview, a letter, a memo, or an e-mail message. Finally, I comment on three errors that nursing students often make in dealing with references: failure to cite the relevant chapter, inappropriate use of secondary sources, and failure to introduce quoted material into the paper in a way that does not break the flow of the narrative.

■ Why Use a Reference?

In preparing an assignment, you may use a number of books, journals, reports, government studies, dissertations, and other materials such as videotapes, items from the popular media such as newspapers and magazines, and information obtained through the Internet. You must acknowledge your indebtedness for the ideas and information you use from these sources. You do this by using a reference or by listing the information in a bibliography.

A reference is used in the body of the paper to show where you use specific information from a specific source; more information about that source is given in the reference list, which usually comes at the end of a paper. A bibliography also comes at the end of a paper, and a listing there indicates only that you read that article, chapter, or book as part of your overall preparation for the paper and therefore are indebted to that source in a general way. A reference also allows readers to consult the sources either to get more detailed information on a point of special interest or to verify your findings if the information seems incorrect or controversial. Thus, you need to indicate how the reader can go about retrieving the original material. You need to tell not only who the expert is but also how to find the material.

Most of your references will likely be to recent books or professional journals, but some of them are hard to find without full details of when and where they were published. Some references (reports, theses, papers presented at conferences) are almost impossible to find without specific information. Because of these difficulties, there are various rules about the way a reference is listed so that a reader can find the information. Style guides or manuals contain these rules (along with other rules, mentioned in earlier chapters of this book, such as when and how to use capitals, how to punctuate, and which dictionary is recommended as a spelling guide).

You use ideas or facts from your reference sources in two ways:

1. You acknowledge that the idea came from another source but para-phrase it (i.e., put the idea in your own words, which must be sub-stantially different from the words used in the original version).
2. You give the idea word for word as a direct quotation.

Either way, you must acknowledge your indebtedness to a source. You need to make it clear that this was not your own original idea but was thought of by someone else. You do this by indicating the source in your paper near the point where it is mentioned; this practice is referred to as "citing the reference."

Plagiarism, which is use of another person's ideas or words without acknowledgment, is a serious offence. In some instances, you may be given a mark of zero for the paper or suspended from the course. You may even be expelled from a college or university for plagiarism. Usually, the calendar of your college or university contains a statement about plagiarism; you should refer to this statement. Many schools of nursing also provide new students with a handout stating the school's position on plagiarism. This is a matter of academic significance, so please take care in citing your references.

The most serious kind of plagiarism, sometimes called complete pla-giarism, is submission of a paper written by someone else for you. Complete plagiarism also includes using the main ideas and large pas-sages from one or more published works as the substance of your paper, even if you paraphrase and acknowledge your sources. Such practices generally represent attempts to cheat.

Using a paper that you wrote for one course for another course is also unacceptable, even if you have modified it and updated the references and content; such a practice is called self-plagiarism. In some instances, you can build a new essay on information developed in an earlier paper, but you should obtain approval from your instructor first and, if requested to do so, provide a copy of the original paper. The new paper must represent more in-depth work, take a new approach, and be significantly different.

A more common instance of plagiarism results from sloppy note-taking during your reading or research or from failing to understand how to acknowledge the material you used from these other sources. Take care when you copy passages from another's work, and distinguish both ideas and phrases used in the original when you make your own statements. Instructors may find it hard to know whether such plagiarism was intentional or accidental.

Information regarded as common knowledge does not have to be supported. For example, if you have spent time in hospitals and been fairly observant, you probably do not need to give a reference for the following idea:

The majority of registered nurses in Canada are married women.

However, if you have relied on specific information taken from another source, you need to identify the source. For example, you probably do not know the exact number of registered nurses who are married, but in a chapter of a book pertinent to this subject you find that Alice Baumgart and Mary Wheeler have done a major study on the nursing workforce in Canada and that they provide statistics on this point. So you might write the following:

About 70% of registered nurses working in Canada are married women (Baumgart & Wheeler, 1992).

Another way of stating this information would be:

Baumgart and Wheeler (1992) report that more than 70% of registered nurses in Canada are married women.

And if you want to use the exact wording from Baumgart and Wheeler, then you must put that information inside quotation marks, as in the following:

Baumgart and Wheeler (1992) report that "in 1990 they [married women] made up more than 70% of the RN work force" (p. 49).

In the examples above, I have used a form of reference called the author-year style, which means that the name(s) of the author(s) and the year of the publication are given within the passage. Then, at the end of the paper, the complete reference information is given in a list organized alphabetically by the names of the authors, usually in a style along these lines:

Baumgart, A. J., & Wheeler, M. M. (1992). The nursing work force in Canada. In A. J. Baumgart & J. Larsen (Eds.), <u>Canadian nursing faces the future</u> (2nd ed.). Toronto: Mosby-Year Book.

The author-year method (which is also called the Harvard method and is the style recommended by the American Psychological Association [APA]) is the one most commonly used in nursing journals in North America. In this method, the writer mentions the authors and the year they published the information in the text; readers who want to know more about the reference look for it in the list at the end under the *authors' names* (or the organization/agency that represents the authors) and the *year*. The author(s) and the year of publication (with a few additional details, such as the author's or authors' initials) are the first two items in each entry in the list.

Methods of citing references vary, often depending on the discipline. For example, English literature tends to use a different style than the social sciences or chemistry. Generally speaking, there are two main styles: use of author-year, and use of numbered references.

You may also see the numerical style used in nursing, and numbered references are the most commonly used style in medical journals and texts. For example, the professional nursing journal of the Canadian Nurses Association, *The Canadian Nurse*, uses the number style. An example of the number style for paraphrasing is the following:

About 70% of registered nurses working in Canada are married women.[1]

If quoting, you would use the numerical style this way:

Baumgart and Wheeler report that "in 1990 they [married women] made up more than 70% of the RN work force."[1]

The list that shows each complete citation is arranged in numerical order, usually at the end of the paper but sometimes at the bottom of each page, and the full citation for the above examples would be something like this (depending on the style recommended for punctuation, capitalization, and so on):

1. Baumgart, A. J., & Wheeler, M. M. The nursing work force in Canada. In A. J. Baumgart & J. Larsen (Eds.), <u>Canadian nursing faces the future</u> (2nd ed.). Toronto: Mosby-Year Book, 1992, p. 49.

When you use a quotation in the author-year style, you indicate the exact source (the page number[s]) in the text of the paper, usually at the end of the sentence; thus, you will have only one mention of each book or article in the reference list at the end of your paper. In the numerical style, the exact source, including the page number(s), is listed numerically at the end of the paper; therefore, if you quote from the same source several times in the paper, you must repeat the citation. To save space when the manuscript is prepared for a journal or book, the second and subsequent mentions are usually given in abridged forms. Some style guides let you repeat the number, but this method can be confusing for both writer and reader when there is a long list of references.

Both the author-year and the numerical styles have strengths and weaknesses. The author-year method allows a knowledgeable reader to assess the importance of a reference without the tiresome chore of flipping to the end of the paper to see if the information comes from a well-known expert or from some esoteric source. As well, the reader can identify how recently the information was published or used; such information is particularly important in research papers. However, when many references are used, the authors' names within the text can be tiresome for the reader. The numerical method is less distracting; the reader can concentrate on the message. The numerical method is particularly useful for short articles, in which readers can quickly find the references.

How do you decide which style to use? Remember to think SMART. Have you been told by your instructor (audience) which style to use? Does the content (message) dictate the style? If you are writing for a newspaper or journal, what style does that publication (route) use? Which style do you (source) prefer? Notice which basic element I asked about first: audience. If your instructor has stated a preference, then you should use that style — or expect to lose marks! Find out if your school of nursing has a preferred style guide; as I noted earlier, APA style is widely used in nursing, and many instructors want students to learn to use it. Check to see if this style is also used in the other departments in your college or university, especially for courses in the humanities or the sciences; other departments may recommend other styles. Many colleges issue a style sheet that all departments are required to follow.

■ A Complete Citation

All style manuals cover much the same material, but the details vary considerably. Fortunately, if you are familiar with one style guide, you can usually find areas of difference in another manual quickly and easily.

The following are the essentials that you need for a complete citation, no matter which style manual you use:

- name(s) of the author(s) of the material;
- year;
- title; and
- information for retrieval.

NAME(S) OF AUTHOR(S)

Your readers will want to be able to identify clearly the author or authors, so you have to note carefully all the names given on the material you read and to note their order. All professions have a few well-known names, and you need to recognize the important ones in nursing. A few style guides require you to use the full first names, but most (including APA) call only for the initials of the first names. But it is a good idea to include the full first names of all authors in your notes because you may need them some day. You will probably be annoyed when you find an important article written by eight or more people, but you do need to list all the authors in your notes. Some style guides allow you to shorten the listing of authors above a certain number, usually more than six. You do this by using the phrase *et al.*, an abbreviation for the Latin *et alii*, which means "and others." If you photocopy pages, be certain to include all the necessary information for a full citation, no matter what the style.

Some style guides require punctuation to be used and the word *and* or an ampersand (&) to be included if there is more than one author; other style guides keep punctuation to a minimum and may omit the *and* or ampersand. This latter style is often used by research journals to save space when there are long lists of references. The following examples show two different styles:

Hibberd, J. M., & Kyle, M. E. (1994). <u>Nursing management in Canada</u>. Toronto: Saunders.

Hibberd JM, Kyle ME (1994). <u>Nursing management in Canada</u>. Toronto: Saunders.

Some style guides recommend that the names of the authors be given in capital letters, which make it easy to see the author and year, or call for a different format so that the names stand out:

HIBBERD JM, and KYLE ME (1994). <u>Nursing management in Canada</u>. Toronto: Saunders.

Styles vary, so you need to select one and learn how to use it properly.

Sometimes a reference book, article, or report is written not by an individual or group of individuals but by an organization or agency. The American Psychological Association in Washington, the Canadian Nurses Association in Ottawa, and the Saskatchewan Lung Association in Regina are examples of organizations that issue publications. For such references, you use the name of the organization as the author. The organization may have produced and distributed the material and is thus also the publisher. For example:

World Health Organization. (1996). <u>Cancer pain relief: With a guide to opiod availability</u>. Geneva: World Health Organization.

Some style manuals, rather than repeat the name of the organization in both places, list it for the author and then use the word *Author* for the publisher, as in the following:

World Health Organization. (1996). <u>Cancer pain relief: With a guide to opiod availability</u>. Geneva: Author.

Be sure that you get the name of the organization right. Students sometimes make mistakes when they mention organizations in the body of the paper. For example, if you refer to "the Social Planning Council's French Language Committee in the Ottawa-Carleton area (1997)," the reader will look for the complete reference in the alphabetical list under "Social"; the reader may then try under "French" and then maybe under "Ottawa." If the reader has to look through the entire list only to find it, eventually, under "Committee on French Language of the Ottawa-Carleton Social Planning Council," he or she may get annoyed. Do you want an annoyed instructor marking your paper?

Sometimes the material was prepared not by an author but by an editor or, in the case of a television program or film, by a director. Usually, this information is given in parentheses after the individual's name and initials, although each style manual has a special method for such listings.

YEAR

In the author-year method, you give the year in which the version of the document that you are using was published. In books, this information is sometimes given on the title page but may only be on the copyright page (which is usually on the back of the title page). Sometimes a book is republished years after it was originally written — and you may need to make this clear in your citation (and in the text). For example, Florence Nightingale's *Notes on Nursing* was written and originally published in 1859, but it has been republished many times since; one such commonly used, widely available facsimile edition was published in 1946. Because it could be confusing to some readers if you indicate 1946 for Nightingale (your readers might think there was another F. Nightingale), you need to make the dates clear in the complete citation. Check the recommended style manual for details of how this should be done. The APA (1994) *Manual* recommends the following style:

Nightingale, F. (1946). <u>Notes on nursing: What it is, and what it is not</u>. Philadelphia: Lippincott. (Original work published 1859)

Another style, not as common, is:

Nightingale, F. (1859/1946). <u>Notes on nursing: What it is, and what it is not</u>. Philadelphia: Lippincott.

If you are using the author-year method and the same author has (or authors have) more than one reference from the same year, you have to add a letter to the year (e.g., 1997*a* and 1997*b*) to distinguish between the items in the paper. For example, if you are using the book *Canadian Nursing Faces the Future*, compiled and edited by Alice J. Baumgart and Jenniece Larsen, you will notice that several other nurses contributed chapters to the book. Each chapter has its own by-line indicating who wrote that material. However, several chapters were written by Baumgart and Larsen themselves. Suppose that you are using material from Chapter 1, entitled "Introduction to Nursing in Canada," and from Chapter 11, entitled (for our purposes) "Inside Nursing Workplaces"; both chapters were written by Larsen and Baumgart (note that for these chapters Larsen is "first author"). The information from Chapter 1 that you paraphrase might go something like this:

> Four major factors affect what Canadian nurses do: professionalism, workplace structure, gender, and change (Larsen & Baumgart, 1992b).

The information that you paraphrase from Chapter 11 might go something like this:

> According to Larsen and Baumgart (1992a), nurses have two major roles, the caregiving role and the co-ordinating role.

Now why did I use the *b* for Chapter 1? This is where it gets complicated! The alphabetical order in the reference list would appear as follows (using APA style for initials, capitals, punctuation, and so on):

> Larsen, J., & Baumgart, A. J. (1992a). Inside nursing workplaces. In A. J. Baumgart & J. Larsen (Eds.), <u>Canadian nursing faces the future</u> (2nd ed.) (pp. 221–238). Toronto: Mosby-Year Book.

> Larsen, J., & Baumgart, A. J. (1992b). Introduction to nursing in Canada. In A. J. Baumgart & J. Larsen (Eds.), <u>Canadian nursing faces the future</u> (2nd ed.) (pp. 3–21). Toronto: Mosby-Year Book.

The reason is that "Inside" precedes "Introduction" in an alphabetical list where the other elements (i.e., authors and year) are the same.

If you fail to use the author-year method correctly, it can be difficult for a reader to find a reference when the list is long — as it would be in a thesis.

TITLE

Even listing a title can be fraught with problems. If you are referencing a book, then give its full title. Frequently, a book is referred to by only a portion of its title (e.g., *Notes on Nursing*), but its full title may have two or more parts (*Notes on Nursing: What It Is, and What It Is Not*). The title should be copied from the title page of the book rather than from the cover because the two sometimes differ; the one on the title page is the correct one.

In the reference list of a student paper, the title of the book is usually underlined, although you (source) may use italics for titles. Underlining is a manuscript convention that dates back to the days of handwriting and typewriters, before computers were common. In any document that was typeset, an italic font was used for book and periodical titles (as well as for names of movies and ships). A writer indicated a title in a manuscript by underlining the words; underlining meant that the words were to appear in print in italics. Thus, style manuals have long recommended to writers (and to students) that the proper way to show titles was by underlining them. The APA (1994) *Manual* recommends underlining because the manual is mainly a guide for writers who are submitting manuscripts to publishers. A student paper, however, is essentially a finished product intended to stand alone, so it may be acceptable to use italics if you (source) wish — and if you have a computer that produces italics easily. In Appendix A of the APA *Manual*, students are advised that, because the paper is the final copy, italics may be used instead of underlining (p. 334). So even if you use the APA *Manual* as a guide for your paper, you (source) can make the decision — if your instructor (audience) allows the use of italics. (In this book, I use underlining for all titles in the reference examples in the text — but note that I use italics for titles within the text; this is a decision that I and my publisher have made.)

The edition number needs to be included as part of the title; the edition number is given on the title page. A first edition is usually not specified, but later editions are. Note that in APA style the title itself is underlined, but the edition number, which you give in parentheses after the title, is not underlined.

If the book is a collection of chapters written by different authors, you need to give both the title of the chapter (not underlined) plus the author(s) or editor(s) and the title of the whole book (underlined). A compilation of chapters by various authors is usually designated as an edited book, and this is normally mentioned on the title page. Look back at the examples from the Baumgart and Larsen book.

If the relevant information is from an article in a journal, then the title of the article is given as well as the title of the journal. Conventions that apply to the publishing world affect the way that this information is listed. For example, the title of the article is not underlined, but the title of the journal is underlined (or put into italics, if this is the style you are using). An example of a complete citation for a typical journal article, using APA style, would be:

Attridge, C. B. (1996). Analysis of powerlessness. <u>Canadian Journal of Nursing Administration, 9</u>(2), 36-59.

When you first begin your nursing course, you may tend to rely on books as references. However, as you proceed through the course, you are expected to do more and more of your reading in professional journals. These periodicals provide the latest information, often newer research that has not yet been included in books. Later, when you are working as a nurse, you will need to read current periodicals to keep abreast of changes in nursing. You therefore need to know how to reference journal materials.

INFORMATION FOR RETRIEVAL

The final item in your full citation is information that enables an interested reader to retrieve your source. This part of the citation used to be called the "publishing information," but with increased use of electronic and on-line resources, "information for retrieval" is a more accurate designation.

The information for retrieval of most books, reports, pamphlets, and other similar published items is fairly simple. The information for serial publications (i.e., journals, magazines, newspapers) differs slightly, as does information required for other forms of references (e.g., films, videotapes, audiotapes, and CD-ROMs).

Retrieval of information obtained on-line is still in its infancy in nursing but is rapidly becoming the way that information will be gathered in the future. It used to take several years for statistical data on the health of large populations, such as rates for Canadian infant mortality and morbidity, to be collected, analyzed, written up, proofread for accuracy, and published. Now agencies such as Statistics Canada can collect and supply such data rapidly, through computers, directly to researchers and health care professionals. So more and more in the future you will need to know how to read other writers' references for on-line materials so that you can retrieve similar information yourself, and you will need to know how to reference the material that you obtain this way so that others can retrieve it. Most style guides, including the APA (1994) *Manual*, still have limited examples of how electronic and on-line data should be referenced, especially by students in courses. However, if you think SMART and have a basic understanding of why references are used and how they are set up, you can probably give most data in a style that will be acceptable to your instructors.

For references to books (and reports and pamphlets), the publishing information includes the name of the publisher (most style guides indicate that it may be shortened) and the city where that publisher has its head office. In the most commonly used style guides, the city comes first, followed by the publisher's name. Some publishers list a number of cities on the title page; usually, only the first one need be used. You should also check for the publisher's address on the copyright page and use the city given with the address there. For example, some publishers have a head office in the United States, but Canadian textbooks from that publisher are issued by the Canadian head office rather than from the American one. This may be so even if the list of cities on the title page starts with the location of the U.S. head office. (This is the case in the Baumgart and Wheeler example used above.)

If the city is well known, you are not required to give the province or state, unless there is likely to be some confusion. For example, a few Canadian publishers are in London, Ontario; you need to distinguish this city from London, England. Almost all style guides now recommend that writers use the standard abbreviations recommended by the post office for province, state, or country. Thus, for London, Ontario, you would use London, ON; you do not need to put London, UK (for United Kingdom), because readers should assume that it is the major world city. You would put Oxford, UK, however, to distinguish it from Oxford, NY (for New York). You also need to think SMART with the cities. If you are writing in Canada for a Canadian audience, then you probably could put Saskatoon, rather than Saskatoon, SK; if you are writing for an American journal, however, you would be wise to designate the province.

How do you get the list of post office abbreviations? Many style guides, including APA, list them. (I made a note in red ink on the inside back cover of my dog-eared copy of the APA *Manual* giving the page number for state abbreviations so that I can find them quickly; I can never remember whether Maine is MA or ME.) You can get a list from the post office and put it on your reference shelf. Your telephone book may also give these designations, usually on the same pages as the area codes.

The city (and province, state, or country abbreviation, if necessary) is usually followed by a punctuation mark (whether it is a comma or a colon depends on the style guide you are following) and then the name of the publisher. Most style guides state that you can use a shortened version of the publisher's name if the publisher is a major one. Thus, you could just put "Merriam" rather than "G. & C. Merriam Company." You will soon catch on to the commonly known nursing textbook publishers. You should take a look at the references and bibliographies in a couple of your nursing textbooks both to see variations in style and to see what kind of information is most commonly used. If the publisher is a small house or a small agency, unknown to the general public, you may also need to give a full address, although this is rare in student papers.

For journals, you do not give the publisher's name and city. Instead, the only publishing information needed is the volume number and the page numbers for the article. As well, if the journal numbers its pages starting with page 1 in each issue, then the issue number (or the month) must also be given. Some journals, usually research publications, number pages consecutively for an entire volume, which usually represents one year's issues of the journal; thus, the first issue (e.g., January) starts with page 1, but the second issue of the same year (e.g., February) could start with page 65 or 149 or some other number, picking up from the previous issue.

The information about the volume and issue is usually given on the cover, in the table of contents, or on the masthead (usually located on or near the table of contents). Some journals give all or part of this information at the bottom of each page. If you photocopy a page or tear out articles for later use, be sure to save all the information needed for your references! Suppose you are using an article entitled "Evidence-Based Nursing Practice: The State of the Art," written by Beverly Simpson and published on pages 22 through 25 in the November-December 1997 issue of the professional journal *The Canadian Nurse: L'infirmière canadienne*. You find on the table of contents page that this is volume 92, issue 10. If you are using APA style, the full reference would look like this:

Simpson, B. (1997). Evidence-based nursing practice: The state of the art. <u>The Canadian Nurse: L'infirmière canadienne, 92</u>(10), 22-25.

One minor point here concerns the name of the journal. The correct name of this journal is *The Canadian Nurse: L'infirmière canadienne*, and in APA style this complete title would be used. In other styles, the title might be abbreviated, for example to *Cdn Nse*. Some instructors accept just *The Canadian Nurse* or even *Canadian Nurse*. You need to think SMART. Would a short version be acceptable to your instructor (audience)? Would it be acceptable to a journal (route)? How do you (source) feel about it?

The publishing information needed for popular magazines is similar to that for professional journals, except that many such magazines do not have volume and issue numbers. If the magazine has volume and issue numbers, use them; if not, put the date the magazine was issued (month and day). Suppose you are using "The Culture of Flowers," written by George Bellows and published on pages 21 and 22 in the November 14, 1997 issue of a weekly magazine called *Surrey Horticulture*. You have checked the cover, the front-page masthead, and the table of contents and cannot find a volume or issue number. If you are using APA style, the full reference would appear like this:

Bellows, G. (1997, November 14). The culture of flowers. <u>Surrey Horticulture</u>, pp. 21-22.

In other author-year styles, it might be given this way:

Bellows, G. (1997). The culture of flowers. <u>Surrey Horticulture</u>, Nov. 14, 1997, pp. 21-22.

The publishing information for newspapers is similar to that for lay magazines.

The publishing information for movies, videotapes, audiotapes, and television programs is generally similar to that for books. If you use these media in preparing your paper, you need to refer to the style manual recommended for your course.

The publishing information for on-line sources (i.e., Internet) usually includes the file information or the Internet address. If you use information obtained from these sources, you need to refer to the recommended style manual for examples of the various routes. You may also wish to discuss citation format with your instructors; some prefer a method that they find easy to use.

Appendix A contains common styles of references, with notes, showing how to use APA style in student papers. The examples will likely suffice for most student papers throughout the first two years of your nursing course. However, you should own (or have easy access to) at least one style manual — and the *Publication Manual of the American Psychological Association*, fourth edition (APA, 1994), is the one most commonly used in nursing today. Between pages 192 and 222, the APA *Manual* gives 77 specific examples of references (e.g., journal, magazine, newspaper, book, pamphlet, report, unpublished typescript, abstract, movie, television show, computer on-line information).

■ Reference List Versus Bibliographic List

Do you know the difference between a reference list and a bibliography? Your style manual may devote several pages to an explanation of this point. The *reference list* (frequently entitled "References" in the subheading) contains all the documents that you have referred to (cited) in the paper. The *bibliography* contains all the documents that you have read to help you understand the content even if you have not actually cited them in the paper.

Thus, you may need two lists at the end of your paper. A bibliography is usually much longer and more complete than a reference list and might include general texts or style guides. If you did not use ideas or information from any books or journals in the body of the paper (highly unlikely for student papers!), you would not even need a reference list. You would, however, want to acknowledge the various books or articles that you reviewed, and so you would have a bibliography.

Graduate students preparing theses (route) definitely need to use both a reference list and a bibliography. Because journals (a different route) usually want to keep the lists in the articles as short as possible, the APA (1994) *Manual* suggests to its audience (remember that this book was prepared for authors writing articles for APA journals) that only a reference list be used. So what about a student paper? Just to complicate matters, the APA *Manual* notes that students may combine the two (see pp. 333–334). The two do not have to be combined, however; you (the source) can decide to use both. In other words, once again you need to think SMART.

Fortunately, the style recommended by APA is the same for either a reference list or a bibliography. Other style guides, though, call for different layouts for the two.

■ Personal Communications

Personal communications include interviews, letters, memos, e-mail messages, and telephone conversations. Usually, they apply to information that you obtained person to person, and they need to be mentioned in a special way within the text of the paper. Because such communications cannot be recovered by your readers, they are not usually listed in the reference list or bibliography; the APA (1994) *Manual* states that they should not be included in the reference list, but other style manuals do recommend a listing. Letters and documents that form part of a historical file in a special collection in a library are always listed, but such a listing often requires a special archival style, so you need to consult a style manual.

For a personal communication to mean something to your readers, you must provide enough information, either in the text or in the reference, to allow them to assess the value of this expert. Suppose that you interviewed a clinical nurse specialist on one of your wards for some information for a paper. The following illustrate two ways that you could identify this expert in the body of the paper:

> A. J. Smith, clinical nurse specialist in the burn unit of Well Known Hospital, said individuals who have severe burns to a large portion of the body suffer profound physical and psychological shock (personal communication, December 5, 1996). She added that it is usually more important to deal with the effects of shock during the emergency period (such as replacement of lost fluids and the emotional distress) than to deal initially with management of the burn wound itself.

> Individuals who have severe burns to a large portion of the body suffer profound physical and psychological shock. Usually, it is more important to deal with the effects of shock (such as replacement of lost fluids and the emotional distress) during the emergency period than to deal initially with management of the burn wound itself (A. J. Smith, clinical nurse specialist, burn unit, Well Known Hospital, personal communication, December 5, 1996).

If you look at the examples only in the APA (1994) *Manual*, my second version appears to be in a different style; you have to read more of the APA *Manual* to discover that my example is correct (and why) — or you need to think SMART.

■ Common Errors in References

Nursing students often make three specific errors when they are doing the references in their papers: failure to cite the relevant chapter, inappropriate use of secondary sources, and failure to introduce quoted material into the paper in a way that does not break the flow of the narrative.

FAILURE TO CITE THE RELEVANT CHAPTER

A number of students make the mistake of referring to a book when they should be referring to a relevant chapter. If the whole book is by a single author or a group of authors, then one reference will do.

However, today many nursing textbooks are compiled by an editor or two and contain chapters written by different authors.

The following is an example of an incorrect reference:

> Some nurse managers may find the participation of staff nurses on management-level committees "threatening" (Baumgart & Larsen, 1992, p. 250).

Although I can refer to this source and check your findings or get further information (the basic purposes of a citation), this is not the way that the author-year method is done. In particular, the APA (1994) *Manual* does not do it this way.

In the example given, Alice Baumgart and Jenniece Larsen are *editors* of a text containing articles (chapters) written either by them or by other *expert authors*. The information in this sentence actually comes from the chapter by Louise Lemieux-Charles and Dorothy Wylie — and they are the ones who should be mentioned in the citation. Thus, the correct way is the following:

> Some nurse managers may find the participation of staff nurses on management-level committees "threatening" (Lemieux-Charles & Wylie, 1992, p. 250).

In the reference list, the full citation would read:

> Lemieux-Charles, L., & Wylie, D. (1992). Administrative issues. In A. J. Baumgart & J. Larsen (Eds.), <u>Canadian nursing faces the future</u> (2nd ed.) (pp. 241-257). Scarborough, ON: Mosby-Year Book.

You may need to give a separate citation for the whole Baumgart and Larsen book in the bibliography (or in a combined references and bibliography listing). The bibliographic mention of the book would indicate that you at least browsed through it and may have read several other chapters that were not specifically referenced. And you may have to list several chapters from the book in the reference list. Doing so may seem to make your reference list longer than necessary, but it represents the correct way to list material from an edited text. This method is clear for your readers, and it gives the credit to the real authors of the information.

CITING SECONDARY SOURCES

Use of secondary sources can create problems in student papers. A secondary source means that you are referring to a text (and its author) cited in another text, but you have not read the original version. *Occasionally*, this is permissible — but students should not do it routinely, and not without good reason. (The fact that you cannot get the original is often an acceptable reason, especially in student papers.)

A main reason you should not use secondary sources is that the primary source (i.e., the author you read) might not have used the original material correctly or might have used it out of context. When you also use it without seeing the original, the error often gets compounded. So either go to the original or cite the material correctly as a secondary source. Another alternative is to word the sentence so that you omit the secondary source altogether and use the primary source as the reference; you have to do this carefully and accurately, of course.

In the reference list, you give the full information only for the secondary source, but you make it clear in the text that you are citing from a secondary source. A good style guide tells you how to do this correctly. You may also need to note when the original work was published. The following illustration might help you to understand this point. In England in 1859, Florence Nightingale wrote: "Bad sanitary, bad architectural, and bad administrative arrangements often make it impossible to nurse." This passage was published the same year in London in a little book called *Notes on Nursing*. This book was republished in the United States in 1860. You may have read a new textbook edited by Judith M. Hibberd and Mavis E. Kyle in which a senior nursing administrator named Mary Pat Skene quoted this passage from Florence Nightingale. In your paper, you might want to use this quotation to illustrate that some common nursing problems have been around for many years — but you cannot get a copy of these rare Florence Nightingale books to check the original source. Thus, you might use Skene's chapter as your secondary source, showing it in your paper this way:

> Nurses have long recognized that poor conditions in the workplace can affect the kind of nursing that can be given. Florence Nightingale, in 1859, recognized these problems, writing that "bad sanitary, bad architectural, and bad administrative arrangements often make it impossible to nurse" (as cited in Skene, 1994, p. 159).

In the reference list at the end of your paper, if you are using APA style, you would then give the following:

Skene, M. P. (1994). Workplace design. In J. M. Hibberd & M. E. Kyle (Eds.), <u>Nursing management in Canada</u> (pp. 159-173). Toronto: Saunders.

You do not have to copy the Nightingale reference from Skene's reference list and put it in your own. Instead, you make it clear in your text that you are referring to a secondary source.

"STICKING IN" QUOTATIONS

Be careful about "sticking in" a quotation, even if you believe that it illustrates your point well. Sometimes you can do it and the reader can immediately understand the logic behind the quotation. Most times, however, you improve the flow of your writing if you "lead in" to the quotation.

Here is a completely fictional example of a poor way to use a quotation:

> Nurses need to be able to communicate well. "All nurses need a master's degree in English grammar" (Zilm, 1923, p. 34). If nurses....

This quotation may mislead the reader. Are *you* advocating that nurses need to have degrees in English but using words from Zilm to back up your idea? The following helps to clear up that question and helps the flow:

> Nurses need to be able to communicate well. Writing fanatic Gwennyth Zilm (1923) even suggested that "All nurses need a master's degree in English grammar" (p. 34). If nurses....

You may have noticed in some books that each chapter starts with a quotation. This literary artifice dates back hundreds of years and is a good creative way to get readers thinking. However, that is a special literary device and usually does not have a place within a paragraph, in which each sentence must flow from one to the other in a way that the reader can follow easily. So when you use a quotation within a paragraph, make it clear how it ties in with the previous sentence.

The same reasoning applies when it comes to including the reference within your paragraph. If you always simply tack it on at the end of the sentence, it may not assist the flow. This is why the author-year method of citation allows writers to put the author's name into the sentence and follow it with the year, as in the two examples above.

■ Summary

As you can see, preparing written assignments can be a tricky business! You need practice to understand how to use references. You may also need some feedback about how you use references so that you can learn to do them better. One way of obtaining such feedback is to exchange a list of references with another student in one of your nursing courses and then spend a few minutes critiquing them for each other. You may be surprised at the number of important points you pick up.

A style manual deals with many minor points. For example, a minor change related to the typing of a manuscript was decided between the third and fourth editions of the APA *Manual*. In the third edition, the APA *Manual* recommended that you should use two spaces after punctuation that ends a sentence; in the fourth edition, it recommended that you should use a single space after punctuation at the end of a sentence. The two spaces after a period was a long-standing tradition taught in typing schools. The use of one space after the period broke with this tradition because computers now set type in a new way. This minor point is something about which you can decide; most instructors will not mark it even if they are relatively strict about other points of APA style. If you type your own papers, however, you may wish to learn this new style.

Exercise 4.1 at the end of this chapter gives you some practice with references and is followed by some feedback that should help you to recognize what to look for when you do references. You may be surprised at what you missed.

Using references correctly is an important part of college- and university-level courses. In this chapter, I have tried to highlight the main reference problems that seem to plague student nurses. I have emphasized use of the *Publication Manual of the American Psychological Association* (APA, 1994). If your school of nursing recommends its use, I urge you to buy a copy and put it beside your dictionary on your reference shelf. Even if your school of nursing recommends another style manual, I suggest that you borrow a copy of the APA *Manual* and spend an evening browsing through this useful reference tool. The APA *Manual* has excellent background chapters on content and organization of your paper, as well as on expression of ideas (writing style and grammar). It also contains material on ethical standards in scientific publication, on ways to present statistics in journal manuscripts, on electronic manuscripts, and on bias in language. Spend a second evening browsing through the manual recommended by your school and you will have an excellent background for writing all your papers now and in the future. Learn how to use the indexes in these manuals so that you can find information quickly when you are finishing the final draft of your paper.

As you do your reading for courses, take a few minutes and look at the writing style of the articles. Learn to read critically for style as well as content. A good style manual will be of use to you throughout your career. Good style is like good nursing — you do not particularly notice it when it is good, but you really notice it when it is bad!

● EXERCISE 4.1 *References*

Just to give you practice doing references and more feedback about specific points to watch, try using both the APA style and the numerical style in the following simple exercise. Imagine that you are writing a paper about students working together on a written assignment and you wish to include as a quotation the sentence "Collaborative research can be fruitful and rewarding." You found this sentence in an article in the February 1991 issue of *The Canadian Nurse*; you look on the table of contents page and find that this is volume 87, issue 2. The two-page article, which appeared on pages 20 and 21, was entitled "Whose Name Comes First?" and the authors were Lan T. Gien and Suzan Banoub-Baddour. The quotation was on page 21. The sentence that you decide to use as a conclusion to your paper is this:

> Although working together on written assignments can be time consuming and frustrating, one article on this subject concluded that "collaborative research can be fruitful and rewarding."

Show how this sentence would be referenced in the text and how the full citation should appear in the list of references at the end of the paper. First try using APA style as described in this chapter and illustrated in Appendix A. Then try using a numerical style.

APA Style
Text Paragraph

Reference Listing

Number Style
Text Paragraph

Reference Listing

● COMMENTS ON EXERCISE 4.1 *References*

Your completed exercises should look something like these. You probably thought of a dozen questions as you began to work on this exercise, so you can see why you need to own a manual — and why managing references is a difficult task!

APA Style
Text Paragraph

Although working together on written assignments can be time consuming and frustrating, one article on this subject concluded that "collaborative research can be fruitful and rewarding" (Gien & Banoub-Baddour, 1991, p. 21).

Reference Listing

Gien, L. T., & Banoub-Baddour, S. (1991). Whose name comes first? *The Canadian Nurse, 87* (2), 20-21.

Some of the points to note here:

- Be sure the page number is given in the parentheses, because this is a direct quotation.
- Watch the position of the period at the end of the text; there are many specific rules, but in this case the period comes after the reference.
- A capital is used only for the first word in the title of the article in the reference listing.
- Capitals are used for all the main words in the name of the journal (a proper name).
- Be sure to lead into the quotation rather than just sticking in the quoted matter; the following is a poor way because it does not lead into the quoted material:

  Although working together on written assignments is difficult, "collaborative research can be fruitful and rewarding" (Gien & Banoub-Baddour, 1991, p. 21).

Number Style
Text Paragraph

Although working together on written assignments can be time consuming and frustrating, one article on this subject concluded that "collaborative research can be fruitful and rewarding."[1]

Reference Listing

1. Gien, Lan T., and Banoub-Baddour, Suzan. "Whose Name Comes First?" The Canadian Nurse, 87, 2, (June 1991), p. 21.

This is only one example of a style using numbers; you may have used another that is acceptable. Some points to note here:

- The reference number used in the text could be in parentheses (1) or in brackets [1] rather than in superscript.
- The page number is not given in the text, only in the reference listing, and not all the page numbers of the article are included in this listing.
- The word *and* is spelled out in this style (& is used in APA style).
- The title of the article is inside quotation marks (some style manuals do not use quotation marks), and the first letters of all main words in the title are capitalized (again, this depends on the style manual).

You cannot learn a style from this exercise or from reading this brief chapter; the subject is too complex. You must practise and keep referring to the chapter or to a style manual. Later in your course, you will likely need a style manual on hand each time you write a major assignment that involves references.

■ References and Recommended Readings

American Psychological Association. (1994). *Publication manual of the American Psychological Association* (4th ed.). Washington, DC: Author.

Buckley, J. (1995). *Fit to print: The Canadian student's guide to essay writing* (3rd ed.). Toronto: Harcourt Brace Canada.

Council of Biology Editors Style Manual Committee. (1994). *Scientific style and format: The CBE manual for authors, editors, and publishers* (6th ed.). New York: Cambridge University Press.

Furberg, J., & Hopkins, R. (1996). *College style sheet* (4th Canadian ed.). Vancouver: 49th Avenue Press/Langara College.

Li, X., & Crane, N. B. (1994). *Electronic style: A guide to citing electronic information.* Westport, CT: Mecklermedia.

Northey, M., & Timney, B. (1995). *Making sense in psychology and the life sciences: A student's guide to research, writing, and style* (2nd ed.). Toronto: Oxford University Press.

The Chicago manual of style (14th ed.). (1993). Chicago: University of Chicago Press.

Webster's standard American style manual. (1985). Springfield, MA: Merriam-Webster.

Submitting a Student Paper

In the shining-up step on the writing PROCESS ladder — the second to last stage, just before typing up or printing out your paper for submission — you ensure that it is presented according to the rules of the route. You need to understand and take care of all the minor details to make this a first-class paper. In this step, as when you were creating the reference list and/or bibliography, you may need to consult a style manual. Here you act as your own copyeditor. As already described in Chapters 1 through 4 (especially in Chapter 2), you will look for consistency in punctuation, spelling, abbreviation, and capitalization. As well, you will check details of presentation, layout, syntax, and style.

In this chapter, I outline the general rules of the route for a formal college- or university-level paper and specifically identify those you must follow in APA style. If you hire a typist for your paper, he or she will already know many of these rules, many of which are standard; you may also want to ask, however, if he or she is familiar with APA style and, if not, go over it to ensure that these details are followed.

Appendix B shows a few pages from a fictional student paper so that you can see how one would look. This appendix can serve as a quick guide to setting up your own paper. The following text includes more explanation about setting up a student paper and gives further examples.

■ General Format

Your assignments should be presented on standard 8.5" x 11", white, unlined paper. You need not buy expensive paper with a high rag content, as is required for some theses and for special business presentations. Use only one side of the sheet. Do not use legal-size (8.5" x 14") paper; the longer pages will make your paper stick out in a pile of assignments and may make it difficult for your instructor to carry and handle them.

Preferably, your final copy should be typed or printed out on a printer of reasonable quality. Dot-matrix printers often produce a typeface that is difficult to read, so ensure that your printer produces a clear, readable typeface. Be sure to have a high-quality ribbon or cartridge that produces sharp, black text in either your typewriter or computer. If you are using a computer or word processor, select a standard typeface, such as Times Roman, Courier, or Pica; these typefaces have tiny lines, called *serifs*, that help to carry a reader's eyes along the line. Typefaces without serifs (called *sans serifs*), such as Helvetica or Gothic and most typefaces on a dot-matrix printer, are more difficult to read and cause readers (including your instructor) to feel tired. (See Box 5.1.) If you are allowed to submit handwritten papers, take care that they are legible. Use black or blue ink; never submit a paper written in pencil.

Whether you submit a handwritten or a typed paper, use margins of at least one inch at the top, bottom, and left and right sides of the page. These standard margins are usually programmed into your word processor or computer, although you can change them. One-inch margins allow your instructor room to write notes and comments on the paper. Occasionally, your instructor will ask you to leave wider margins so that he or she can provide more feedback. As always, an instructor's special requirements override all other style guidelines.

BOX 5.1 *Serif and Sans Serif Fonts*

Courier is a typeface with serifs.
Letter Gothic is a sans serif typeface.

Always double-space lines (even for handwritten papers) in the body of the paper; doing so makes it easy to read. Because your paper is a finished product in itself, and not a manuscript being submitted to a publisher for typesetting, you may choose to use single spacing for some parts of your paper. Appendix A of the *Publication Manual of the American Psychological Association* (APA, 1994, pp. 331-340) advises that you may use single spacing in tables, footnotes, and long quotations. You may also use single spacing in your references and/or bibliography (although you must then double-space between entries to make it easy for the reader to see each one separately). Generally speaking, double spacing in the reference lists is easier to read, so you may want to use it there as well. You may also choose to use triple spacing before subheadings and in other places where it would improve the appearance of your paper (e.g., on the title page, after a title or a table, and before footnotes, or to avoid having a subheading on the bottom line of a page).

Number your pages in the top right-hand corner, using arabic numbers, beginning with the title page. You should also use an identifying header at the top right-hand side of the page either immediately above or five spaces to the left of the page number. These headers are useful in case pages of an assignment become separated during marking or mixed with another student's paper. A header usually consists of the first two or three words of the title of your paper. You should avoid using your name as the header (unless your instructor requests otherwise); some instructors prefer to mark papers without knowing the student's name, and later in your career, when you submit articles to journals, they are reviewed anonymously. You may choose to omit the page number on the title page of a student paper if you believe that doing so will improve the appearance — even if you are following APA style. If you use a computer, learn to set headers and page numbers automatically; such a learning investment will save you hours of reformatting!

Indent the first line of every paragraph and the first line of references and footnotes five to seven spaces; on a typewriter or computer, this is best done using the tab key. Certain passages in the text, such as long quotations (i.e., block quotations) and some lists, may also need to be indented; this is best done using the indent key or keys.

Even if you do not intend to master the computer keyboard, you should learn basics related to typing and setting margins, tab keys, indent keys, underlining, and bold type; these functions can save you hours of work when it is necessary to edit or reformat your papers.

Remember, formats differ for other routes. For example, if you are writing a paper for a journal that uses APA style, the finished version can be transmitted on disk or electronically rather than as a hardcopy manuscript. In that kind of manuscript, no bold type is used (even for headings).

■ Headings

Headings are another matter of style that may differ in student papers. The APA (1994) *Manual* describes five levels of headings that may be necessary in articles. These are guidelines, and an author may select the level of heading that most suits the content of the article. The first four levels recommended by APA for manuscripts submitted to APA journals are shown in Box 5.2.

BOX 5.2 *Headings*

Level One Headings

This is the primary heading that would be used, for example, for the title of the article. It is usually used only once in an article. Notice that it is centred and that the initial letters of the main words are capitalized. In student papers, this heading could be set in boldface. Bold letters are not used in manuscripts submitted to journals using APA format because editors determine the font that should be used for the title; think about articles that you have seen in journals and you will recall that many of these titles are set in large type.

Level Two Headings

Level two headings are centred and underlined. Notice that the initial letters of all main words are capitalized. Note also that there is no extra line of space (i.e., a quadruple space) between the sections in the article.

Level Three Headings

The third level is set at the left-hand margin of the page above the indented paragraph and is underlined. Again, initial letters are capitalized, and no extra line of space is used.

Level four headings. This level is also known as a paragraph heading. It is indented (using the tab key) the same distance as a paragraph, and the remaining part of the paragraph continues. Notice the sentence-type capitalization.

The APA *Manual* says that four levels of headings should be enough for most articles. In some special research papers or in a thesis, a fifth level may be necessary; in these cases, you should follow the style manual.

Notice that some text follows each heading; only rarely are headings set together without some intervening text. Usually, two subheadings follow one another only within tables.

Fortunately, most student papers are relatively short and need only two or three levels of headings. You may also decide to use extra line spaces before headings and to put the headings into **bold** or <u>underlined</u> type to make them stand out. For example, you could set your headings as shown in Box 5.3.

■ Parts of a Student Paper

When formatting your paper, consider if you have included all the parts that may be required. Usually, each part starts on a separate page. A formal student essay may contain some or all of these elements:

- cover page (or title page);
- table of contents or outline page;
- abstract;

BOX 5.3 *Alterations to Headings*

Right Ways to Write:
Better Papers Mean Better Grades

Your introductory paragraphs would come here. Note that you would not put the subheading "Introduction" immediately below the title. APA makes this recommendation because it avoids two headings coming together and because it should be obvious, without the label, that the opening paragraphs actually are the introduction. The omission of this heading also allows journal editors to save a couple of lines of space.

<u>First Level Heading in Right Ways</u>

This heading might be the first major one in the body of your paper and one of the three in your outline. In most papers, it would be the only heading you need.

- text of paper (but remember that the text of a student paper almost always contains an introduction, body [with its two, three, or four main parts], and conclusion);
- references;
- bibliography;
- appendix or appendices.

Many student papers, especially first-year papers, need only a cover page, the main text, and a reference list (or combined references and bibliography). On the other hand, a master's thesis requires a title page, approval page, acknowledgments, table of contents, lists or tables and/or figures, abstract, body of the thesis (usually divided into several chapters), appendices, and separate references and bibliography; it may also include a foreword and a preface, which come before the main body of the thesis, and an index, which comes at the end.

How do you determine what is needed? First, check the course syllabus for instructions about the assignment; most instructors state their requirements there. If you are in doubt, ask during one of the classes.

Usually, a table of contents or outline of the paper is not required. However, many nursing instructors ask first-year students to submit one or the other because instructors know the importance of the **O** in PR**O**CESS; they want students to get into the habit of **o**rganizing their papers. Furthermore, if your ideas do not move smoothly from one section to another, a table of contents or outline helps the instructor to see your overall plan.

An abstract is a comprehensive summary of your paper — usually only 100 to 120 words long, though some have restrictions of 75 to 100 words. An abstract is an essential component of most journal articles; it provides a capsule statement that tells readers what your article is about, what your conclusions are, and how these findings can be interpreted. Its main purpose is to assist readers when they do literature searches and must review hundreds of articles. This brief statement can appear alone (e.g., in an on-line summary, or in a journal containing abstracts related to a particular subject); potential readers can usually tell from the abstract whether they wish to obtain and read the whole article. The APA (1994) *Manual* devotes a section to describing what an abstract is, and some instructors, particularly those in more senior years, ask students to write them as a learning experience.

An abstract differs from an introduction (even if you write an abstract, you still need an introduction to the body of your paper), although the two are similar in content. A main difference is that an abstract includes a summary of the findings, whereas an introduction indicates where the article is going and does not necessarily reveal all the findings. For theses, a special kind of abstract is often written before the writer begins the research that will be described in the paper. There are different kinds of abstracts for different messages. For example, abstracts submitted to conference review committees are usually longer and are often written before the paper is prepared. Students, however, usually find it best to write the abstract after the body of the paper is in its final draft.

■ Important Pages

Formatting the cover page and the first page of your paper is of special importance. This section discusses in detail how to format these pages. For further examples and for examples of other pages, see Appendix B. These examples are intended only as guides. For your own papers, remember to think SMART.

COVER PAGE

One of the most important items in the final draft of your paper is a good cover page or cover sheet. Sometimes called a title page, it goes at the front of your assignment — but it differs from the title page of an article being submitted to a journal. And, unlike the abstract, it is often a good idea to work on your title page — or at least on the title itself — as soon as you begin to plan your paper.

The cover page of the student paper usually differs from the style described in detail in the APA (1994) *Manual*; remember that a student paper is a different route than an article and that the requirements are different. And, because the student paper is the end product, you (source) can make your own decisions — provided you consider the content needed (message) and your instructor (audience) has not given specific instructions.

On the final draft of the cover page (during the shining-up stage), you should include some basic information: the title of your paper, your name, your student number, the name of the course (and section, if the course is divided into sections), the name of the university, and your instructor's name. If you are taking the course through a distance education program, your address is also essential. Inclusion of your address is a sound idea for on-campus students as well, because occasionally an instructor needs to mail back an assignment (e.g., the final assignment of the year). You may wish to include your phone number; some instructors may phone to comment on your paper or provide additional feedback if you make it easy for them.

A catchy title is a great idea. It introduces your assignment and can provide, in a brief phrase or two, a capsule comment on your topic. The title should be clear and interesting. You may also want to include a subtitle. For example:

Right Ways to Write:
Better Papers Mean Better Grades

Some instructors provide you with information in the course syllabus on what they want or expect on the cover sheet. If your instructor does so, then follow that style.

You may wish to develop your own style for the cover page. Just be sure to include all the essentials. And, even if you are a wonder on the computer and can develop a cover with different, large, beautiful fonts and borders, remember that this is a student paper, not a document for sale. Fancy typefaces and graphics may give a different tone than you intended; some instructors do not like to receive a paper that looks as if you spent more time designing the cover than working on the content!

A sample cover sheet — a plain, simple one — is shown in Box 5.4. This version does not use single spacing anywhere, but it does use quadruple spacing. It does not use the running head and the page number (although this is page 1), but it does identify the running head that will be used in the rest of the paper. You may decide to format your cover differently, perhaps using single spacing for the address, but this style is offered as a model.

FIRST PAGE OF BODY OF PAPER

The following example (Box 5.5) of the first page of a student paper is based on the APA (1994) *Manual* but allows a few modifications suitable in a student paper. The difference between this modified style (for a student paper) and pure APA style (for an article to be sent to a journal; see Box 5.6) is that the title is set two spaces down and put in

BOX 5.4 *Sample Cover Sheet*

RIGHT WAYS TO WRITE:
Better Papers Mean Better Grades

by Glennis Zilm
Student Number: 98-7654321

Running head: Right Ways

Assignment #1 (September 8, 1998)
Writing Skills Course E107x
University of Surrey

Instructor: Cheryl Entwistle, RN, BSN, MEd

Glennis Zilm
#306 — 1521 Blackwood St.
White Rock, B.C. V4B 3V6
Phone: 535-3238

BOX 5.5 *Sample Essay Beginning*

Right Ways   2

Right Ways to Write:
Better Papers Mean Better Grades

   Students who follow style guides carefully when they submit their papers are more likely to receive higher marks. Although instructors are most concerned with the content of a paper, appearance does affect how they read. Style can make reading easy or difficult; instructors (who read hundreds of papers a year) like the reading to be easy so that they can concentrate on the content and provide feedback to the student.

BOX 5.6 *Sample Pure APA Style*

....

Right Ways   2

Right Ways to Write:
Better Papers Mean Better Grades

Students who follow style guides carefully when they submit their papers are more likely to receive higher marks. Although instructors are most concerned with the content of a paper, appearance does affect how they read. Style can make reading easy or difficult; instructors (who read hundreds of papers a year) like the reading to be easy so that they can concentrate on the content and provide feedback to the student.

---

immediately after the cover page; that is, there are no table of contents and no abstract.

■ Checklist for Final Typing of Student Papers (APA Style)

....

The following checklist reviews some of the points you need to keep in mind when shining up your paper.

- Use white copy paper, size 8.5" x 11".
- Set at least one-inch margins at top, bottom, and left and right sides of all pages.
- Justify the left margin, but leave the right margin unjustified ("ragged").
- Use a standard typeface with serifs, such as Times Roman, CG Times, Courier, or Pica.
- Double-space lines in the main text (and in most other parts of the paper *unless* other spacings would improve appearance and readability).
- Number all pages in the top right-hand corner beginning with the title page.
- Identify your running head on the cover page and set it to appear on each page of your paper either five spaces to the left of the page number or immediately above the page number.
- Read the paper aloud: is it easy to read, or do you stumble any-

where?
- Check the length of your sentences: are there too many long sentences?
- Do too many sentences start the same way? Look especially for sentences with weak openings such as "There are ... " or "This is ... " or "It was...."
- Check for improper use of first-person pronouns (I, we, my, our, me, ours).
- Have you used jargon, slang, or clichés?
- Are too many sentences in the passive voice?
- Check the style of your title, headings, and subheadings.
- Check the spelling of any word about which you are not completely certain; if you use a computer and have a spell checker, learn how to use it.
- Check the use of capitals: are they consistent? Do you have a reason for using the capital letters you used throughout your paper?
- Check the punctuation: have you used a comma before the word *and* in a series of three or more items? Do you have too many commas? Are there quotation marks where they are needed? Have you used apostrophes appropriately? Are there too many dashes and exclamation points (which signal an informal tone)?
- Give your paper to your typist — and when you get it back, proofread it through a final time; do not change your content, but make any minor corrections neatly in black ink on the final version.
- Keep a photocopy of your paper; even the best instructors occasionally misplace a paper.
- *Always remember that your instructor's requirements outrank all other style guidelines.*

■ Submitting the Paper

Finally, you are ready to submit your paper. Most instructors prefer to get the paper without an envelope or cover; some prefer an envelope, especially if the paper is to be returned by mail, or a cover to help keep papers separate from one another during marking. APA guidelines advise that you submit the paper with a paperclip in the top left corner, rather than stapled; this makes it easier for both editors and instructors, who sometimes like to spread the paper out and look at various pages at the same time (e.g., the body of the paper and the references).

Try to submit the paper on time, unless you have a good reason for a delay. If you need an extension, ask for one rather than just submit the paper late.

Two self-assessment exercises that review points to look for in the shining-up step are included here. Try them.

● **EXERCISE 5.1** *Grammar, Usage, Spelling, and Punctuation*

This short paragraph contains errors in grammar, usage, spelling, and punctuation. See how many you can spot and correct.

In order to efficiently apply for most senior positions, resumes should be used. Potential applicants often seek advise from communication experts in designing their résumés, however some of the suggestions from these consultents are a bit flamboyant and they are unsuited to conservative health care institutions. All recommendations should be weighed carefully. Noone should accept poor council which may effect their futures.

● **COMMENTS ON EXERCISE 5.1** *Grammar, Usage, Spelling, and Punctuation*

1. Change *In order to efficiently apply* to *To apply* (unnecessary words).
2. Delete *most* (unnecessary).
3. Change *resumes* to *résumés* (check spelling and Canadian usage in *Gage Canadian Dictionary* [de Wolf, Gregg, Harris, & Scargill, 1997] and be consistent throughout the paper; note that the spelling in the next sentence is résumés).
4. Change *résumés should be used* to *applicants should use résumés* (résumés do not apply for senior positions — applicants do; poor sentence and passive voice).
5. Change *Potential applicants* to *Many job hunters* (clarity; shorter words; prevents repetition of applicants in the rewritten version).
6. Change *advise* to *advice* (either a misused word or a typing error).
7. Change *in designing their résumés* to *about résumé design* (ambiguous pronoun reference; *their* could refer to experts or to applicants).

8. Change the comma to a semicolon before *however* and insert a comma after *however* (original is a "run-on sentence"; alternative: change the comma to a period and start the next sentence with *However* and a comma).

9. Delete *of the* (unnecessary).

10. Change *consultents* to *consultants* (either a spelling mistake or a typing error; tighten the sentence by removing *a bit*, a lazy and vague modifier, then reword latter part of sentence both to remove the pronoun *they*, which could refer to *consultants*, and to reduce the length of the sentence).

11. Change *All recommendations should be weighed carefully* to *Weigh recommendations carefully* (removes passive voice).

12. Change *Noone* to *No one* (either a spelling mistake or a typing error).

13. Change *council* to *counsel* (misuse of word).

14. Change *which* to *that* (misuse of word).

15. Change *effect* to *affect* (misuse of word).

16. Change *their futures* to *his or her future* (lack of agreement; pronoun[s] must agree in number with *No one*; alternative: change *their futures* to *one's future*).

The following is the revised, polished version (48 words compared with 62 words in original; average number of words per sentence 12 compared with 15.5 in original; one long sentence with 23 words compared with one long sentence with 33 words in original):

> To apply for senior positions, applicants should use résumés. Many job hunters seek advice from communication experts about résumé design; however, suggestions from some consultants may be unsuitable for health care professionals. Weigh recommendations carefully. No one should accept poor counsel that may affect his or her future.

● **EXERCISE 5.2** *Shining Up the Final Copy*

The following exercise reviews the kind of shining up you should do in your final review.

1. Delete extraneous words in the following sentences.
- He is in the process of drawing up the nominations.
- She intends to take action without further delay.

2. Polish the following poor sentences.

- She did not think that it was unimportant to wear neat, professional dress.
- The union was not unwilling to negotiate on the offer.
- Well Known Hospital (WKH) will be responsible for the development and execution of a health promotion day designed to increase awareness in the local community about WKH's Wellness Clinic.

3. Think about the double meanings in the following sentences.

- Yesterday, the police tied the suspect to the car used in the holdup.
- New mothers find it much harder to manage when they have children.

● COMMENTS ON EXERCISE 5.2 *Shining Up the Final Copy*

1. Following are shorter, clearer versions.

- He is drawing up the nominations.
- She intends to take action now.

2. The following are improved versions.

- She thought that neat professional dress was important. (This version avoids double negatives.)
- The union was willing to negotiate on the offer.
- Well Known Hospital will develop and carry out a health promotion day to inform the local community about its Wellness Clinic.

OR

- Well Known Hospital will develop and carry out a health promotion day to help make the local community aware of its Wellness Clinic.

3. You could rewrite these sentences several ways, if you have time. The two humorous examples should remind you that sometimes you get too close to your work — although a sentence makes good sense to you, it may not make good sense to your readers.

■ Summary

These five chapters have described in detail the writing PROCESS for a student paper. This chapter concentrated on the rules for formatting a student paper. Please do not be overwhelmed by what seem to be so many rules; soon they will come almost automatically if you practise them. During your student days, you may write 50 or more papers, so learning the rules early and reviewing them often will pay off in the long run.

Appendices A and B contain examples to which you will likely need to refer fairly often, especially when preparing papers early in your student career. If you go on into the final years of a degree course or into graduate school, you will likely need to supplement this book with the style manual recommended by your school of nursing. Appendix C contains an annotated list of reference tools that may be helpful to you as you proceed through your career and become even stronger as a writer.

I want to stress that you should think SMART in every written communication that you prepare. After reading this far in the book, you should be a much more informed source than you were and should have a much better idea of your strengths and weaknesses. You should realize that you need good writing tools to assist you. You will need to work hard on the message of each new paper; most of that content will come from the courses you take and the readings and materials assigned for them. You should be much more aware of the importance of your audience, who for student papers is the instructor or, sometimes, a designated marker; students who ask questions and discuss feedback are usually much more successful than those who do not. You should now have a much better understanding of the route (student paper) and appreciate that it has many rules, but it also has maps (or style guides). And you should now understand how tone affects your writing and realize that student papers are a relatively formal method of presentation.

The next chapter describes other routes that you will use during your nursing career. You may not need to read that chapter for a while, although if you read it now you will find that it reviews and reinforces many of the principles behind The SMART Way to approach all written communications.

Writing is, and probably always will be, hard work — but so are many other enjoyable activities, such as gardening, mountain climbing, or hockey. Look upon this learning experience as a challenge that will pay off and make your future more enjoyable. The writing skills that you practise now will benefit you later in your nursing career. Good luck in your writing!

■ References

American Psychological Association. (1994). *Publication manual of the American Psychological Association* (4th ed.). Washington, DC: Author.

de Wolf, G. D., Gregg, R. J., Harris, B. P., & Scargill, M. H. (1997). *Gage Canadian dictionary*. Vancouver: Gage Educational Publishing.

SMART Ways for
Other Routes
in Nursing

The SMART elements of communication and the steps in the writing PROCESS will work for you throughout your career. Once you have practised using them and have learned the basics related to each type of written communication, you should be able to master each new route fairly quickly. In this chapter, I go over the fundamentals of a variety of routes — business letters, memos, e-mail, résumés, reports, and articles — that you will meet in your career. Each one requires practice, of course, and you can learn and apply numerous details for each type of communication; in fact, there is at least one book devoted to each of the routes described in this chapter. But if you think SMART and draw on the basics from earlier in this book, you should adapt well to all routes.

■ Business Letters

You learned the fundamentals of business letters in grade school and have probably already had to write a number of business letters. For example, many schools of nursing require that you write a formal letter of application, which is one type of business letter. During your course, you may also need to communicate formally with your school of nursing or with an instructor, and you may need to use a business letter to do that.

Basically, all letters have much the same form. As the writer of the letter, you are the source. Even if you are sending much the same message (e.g., "I am applying for a job"), each audience (e.g., friend, personnel officer) is likely different. Even if you are a friend of the individual to whom you are sending a business letter, you treat it differently because it is not just sent to that individual but may become part of the office or agency files. The main differences between a personal letter (i.e., one you would send to a friend) and a business letter apply to a few rules of route and a distinct difference in tone. However, even business letters can have differences in tone, from highly formal to informal but still businesslike.

Almost all business letters are done on stationery that is 8.5" x 11". The paper should be of good quality and be either a basic white or a neutral, formal color (cream, grey, pale blue) and should have business-size envelopes (9" x 4" or 9.5" x 4") that match in color. Letters are folded into three to fit into these envelopes. You can get colored and printed (e.g., floral) stationery in these sizes (mainly because they fit into computer printers easily), but save them for personal letters.

Should a business letter always be typed? You need to think SMART and work out your own answer to that question. For example, when you are just starting out to find employment, you may not have much money, and paying a typist to type letters of application to potential employers can be costly. If you write neatly and legibly, a short, handwritten letter of application that accompanies a typed résumé will probably be acceptable to most hospital or agency personnel offices; some potential employers like to see your handwriting because it often reveals details about you (e.g., whether you can spell!). On the other hand, if you are writing an application asking for several thousand dollars of funding for equipment on your unit, then you would be wise to use a well-qualified secretary employed by the agency to do the layout. If you are writing a letter of thanks to the president of the volunteers on behalf of your unit, a legible, handwritten note on hospital stationery would usually be acceptable and might convey a warmer, more friendly tone than a typed letter. If, on behalf of the staff of your unit, you are writing a letter of condolence to the family of a former patient, a handwritten formal note might be the most appropriate format, even though this communication might be classified as a business letter.

BASIC FORMAT OF A BUSINESS LETTER

As you may remember from your school days, the basic format for a business letter is

- address or letterhead;
- date;
- file numbers (optional);
- inside address (complete name and address of the individual and company to whom you are writing, including all details, such as postal code);
- reference line(s) (optional; may go below the salutation);
- salutation (the "Dear ..." line, sometimes optional);
- body of letter (in which you use the outline);
- complimentary close;
- signature;
- typed name (sometimes optional; e.g., it would be omitted if you use your own letterhead);
- stenographic reference (writer's initials/typist's initials); and
- note regarding enclosures or copies.

Boxes 6.1 and 6.2 show the basic format for two relatively simple business letters. The first is set in a style known as "flush left," which has been adopted by many businesses in recent years; all new sections of the letter, including paragraphs, start at the left-hand margin. The second letter follows a more traditional indented style and is suitable for handwritten business letters. If you have access to the services of a typist or typing pool, you can usually leave the decisions about layout of the business letter to her or him. If you type your own business letters, follow the flush left style, because it is by far the easiest to set up. Instructors at secretarial schools teach rules about setting up the spacing between the various sections, but if you have to do the spacing yourself, then position the letter in the centre of the page and leave double spaces between sections. Some of these basic parts deserve a few additional comments — especially because some of the comments apply to other routes, such as memos and e-mail messages.

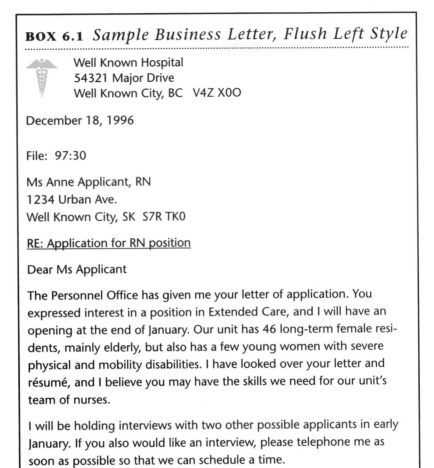

BOX 6.1 *Sample Business Letter, Flush Left Style*

Well Known Hospital
54321 Major Drive
Well Known City, BC   V4Z X0O

December 18, 1996

File: 97:30

Ms Anne Applicant, RN
1234 Urban Ave.
Well Known City, SK S7R TK0

RE: Application for RN position

Dear Ms Applicant

The Personnel Office has given me your letter of application. You expressed interest in a position in Extended Care, and I will have an opening at the end of January. Our unit has 46 long-term female residents, mainly elderly, but also has a few young women with severe physical and mobility disabilities. I have looked over your letter and résumé, and I believe you may have the skills we need for our unit's team of nurses.

I will be holding interviews with two other possible applicants in early January. If you also would like an interview, please telephone me as soon as possible so that we can schedule a time.

The best times to reach me are weekday afternoons between 1300 and 1500 hours. Telephone the hospital number above and ask for local 305.

Sincerely

Kerin Smithers, RN, BSN
Unit Care Manager
Westbrook Unit

KS/at

Copy: Personnel Office, T. K. Paterson

BOX 6.2 *Sample Business Letter, Indented Style*

Well Known Hospital
54321 Major Drive
Well Known City, BC   V4Z X0O

December 18, 1996

Mrs. R. K. Helper, President
 WKH Auxiliary
  c/o 123 Country Ave.
   Well Known Suburb, AB T7K R8O

Dear Mrs. Helper

 On behalf of Westbrook Extended Care Unit, I wish to thank you for the two new Ezy-Lift chairs donated this month by the Auxiliary. These two chairs are valuable for assisting arthritic elderly residents get to their feet with a minimum of nursing assistance. One resident told me this morning how much she likes the chair and how much safer she feels.

 WKH Auxiliary has done so much for our Hospital, and I want you to know how much your gifts are appreciated by residents and staff. Please, the next time you are at the hospital, drop by the unit, and I will arrange to show you how delightfully the chairs fit into the sun porch.

 Please extend our thanks to all members of your group.

                              Sincerely

                              (Ms) Kerin Smithers, RN
                              Unit Care Manager
                              Westbrook Unit

ADDRESS OR LETTERHEAD

If you are writing a business letter on behalf of your employer, you would use the letterhead of the hospital, agency, or company; you are acting as a source on behalf of that agency. The letterhead contains the return address, and all mail in reply to your letter would be sent to that address. You may need to add a typed line immediately below to indicate how mail should be directed to you within the agency (e.g., the name of the ward).

You would almost never use a company letterhead and ask for a reply to be sent to you at another address (e.g., your home address), although there are a few exceptions (e.g., when you write on behalf of a club or association and wish to speed up mail delivery); you need, however, to make this point clearly in the body of the letter.

You may also need to write business letters from your home on your own behalf (e.g., to apply for a job, to write to a politician or a newspaper stating an opinion, or to ask for a correction to a bank document). In today's world of computers, you may wish to develop your own letterhead, as shown in Box 6.3. Save your letterhead on a disk or your hard drive so that you can use it whenever you write a business letter. You can also buy a printed letterhead for yourself (expensive) or hire a secretarial service to type up and run off a few dozen copies for you to use (much less expensive). Such letterheads are not difficult to design, but you do need to keep a few SMART principles in mind as you do so. For business, the letterhead should be slightly formal; plain is generally better than fancy — but you can think SMART. For example, Madonna might select a more daring letterhead if she were writing to a producer to line up a job than you would choose if you were writing to a public health department asking for a staff position. If you (source) weigh the message, audience, and tone, you should be able to design a personal business letterhead that is creative and suitable.

BOX 6.3 *Sample Personal Letterheads*

....

GLENNIS ZILM

P.O. Box 71513 Hillcrest Post Office
1453 Johnston Road, White Rock, B.C. V4B 3Z0
Telephone (604) 535-3238 E-mail Glennis1@aol.com

- - - - - - - - - - - - - - - -

GLENNIS ZILM
#306—1521 Blackwood St., White Rock, B.C. V4B 3V6

INFORMATION BEFORE THE BODY OF THE LETTER

Many individuals wonder whether they should write December 22, 1996 or 22 December 1996 or some other version for the date of the letter. I like the former, with the month spelled out, but you can use the format you want. You might want to note that health care agencies tend to use the international format (the latter version).

A file number is only necessary in a large agency, such as a hospital, and you have to learn the method used. A file number might be used on job applications, as in the sample letter shown in Box 6.1. If you are responding to a letter that used a file number, you should quote that number in any further correspondence. For example, if Anne Applicant responded to Kerin Smithers, she would put in this line:

Your file number: 97:30

The inside address is an essential part of a business letter and should be as complete as possible. For best results, you should always attempt to find out the name of an individual to whom to address your letter (although this information is not always available). For example, if you are writing a letter to the editor of a professional journal, you should check a recent copy of the journal and find out the name of the editor. If you are sending a job application to a small hospital or agency in your area, you may want to telephone the switchboard and ask to whom the letter should be addressed; you may not want to do this if it involves a costly long distance call. If you are writing to a large urban hospital, where there are likely several individuals working in the department, you could address the letter to the Personnel Office or the Human Resources Department). Remember, however, that almost any reader likes to be addressed by name.

Using a name for the inside address is also helpful in writing the salutation; you then address the individual by name. Thus, you do not have to use the completely out of date "To Whom It May Concern" or the old-fashioned "Dear Sir or Madam"; some recipients find these salutations (especially the latter) offensive. Many letter writers worry about how to write the salutation when they have only the initials of the individual or have a first name for a woman but do not know whether to write "Ms," "Mrs.," or "Miss." My advice to these worriers is to concentrate on writing a good message in the body of the letter. Then simply think SMART about the details of the salutation. If you do find out the name, also try to find out if it belongs to a Mrs. or Miss or Dr. You can also use the first name or initials with the last name if that is the way the person has signed a letter to you (e.g., "Dear Mary Jones" or "Dear M.T. Jones"). If you do not have a name, you can omit the salutation altogether and just use a reference line. (See sample letters in Appendix C.)

The reference line usually highlights the subject of the letter (as in the example in Box 6.1). You can use "RE:" or "Re:" or "Subject:". The reference line is usually underlined, but some sources prefer to use all capital letters. A reference line might also be used to highlight something important, such as "<u>Personal and confidential</u>."

Some style guides for business letters say that you can use the reference line to bring the letter to the attention of some individual within the company, as in the following example.

Personnel Office
Well Known Hospital
54321 Major Drive
Well Known City, BC   V4Z X0O

ATTENTION: Mary Jones, Personnel Officer

Dear Ms Jones

This kind of address might be used if you had spoken to Mary Jones on the phone before you sent the letter but wanted it to convey the message that you were not writing to her personally but sending a general letter of application.

INFORMATION AFTER THE BODY OF THE LETTER

The complimentary close comes immediately after the body of the letter, separated by a double space. The complimentary close most commonly used now in business letters is "Sincerely," although some companies use "Yours truly." Some complimentary closings are long outdated, such as "Your faithful servant." (And, after reading Chapter 3 in this book, you would never use "Very truly yours," would you?) If you have had a long business correspondence with an individual or have come to know the person, you might want to alter the closing for that individual and use something like "Best wishes."

After the complimentary close, you leave some space for your signature. For business letters to someone you do not know, you should generally avoid using nicknames or diminutives and develop a consistent signature (e.g., Marjorie Jones rather than Marj Jones). Once you know the correspondent well, you may elect to sign with the name that she or he calls you (e.g., Marj). You do not write in your courtesy title (e.g., Mrs.), your degree(s) (e.g., RN), or your title (e.g., Unit Manager).

The typed signature line goes below your signature — even if the latter is legible. This line does contain the courtesy title, degree(s), and title; you may need an extra line if your job title is long. Make it clear in the typed signature how you wish to be addressed. For example, you may sign the letter "Nancy Nadon," but the typed signature might read "(Mrs.) Nancy Nadon, R.N." or "Nancy Nadon, RN (Miss)."

If you type your own letter, you do not need a stenographic reference. If a secretary types the letter, he or she will put in your initials followed by his or her own.

If you are adding enclosures to the letter or sending a copy of the letter to some other person or department, make a note to this effect by adding the accepted abbreviations for enclosure (enc) or carbon copy (cc).

HELPFUL HINTS FOR THE BODY OF THE LETTER

Although I have taken a number of pages to go over the rules of the route for letters, always remember that the message in the body of the letter is the most important part. The ways to develop a good body of a letter are the same as those already described in Chapters 1 through 5. First of all, think SMART.

Keep in mind who you (source) are and why you are writing. If you are writing on behalf of your employer, be aware that what you say and how you say it will reflect on your employer (and ultimately on your job). Sometimes (as in the example of the letter to the president of WKH Auxiliary) you are writing on behalf of those who work for you.

Work out what your message really is; you may even want to summarize it in the reference line so that it will be at the top of the letter. Your message should be presented in the same three-part outline that works for assignments. The opening paragraph, which should be short, is the introduction and tells the individual what the letter is about. The body of the message is conveyed in the next paragraph or two (or more if necessary). The final paragraph, which also should be short, is the conclusion and should sum up what you want the recipient of the letter to do. Like the conclusion to a student paper, the final paragraph or sentence will stay in the reader's mind, so it should be positive, interesting, stimulating, and creative. Depending on the importance of the letter, you may want to spend extra time on the beginning and ending as well as on the important basic information in the middle. If you are writing a letter to your mother, she will likely be so delighted to hear from you that you can open with a trite remark such as "How are you? I am fine" and close with "Give my love to dad, and ask him to send me an extra five dollars for a pizza." On the other hand, if you are writing a letter to all the graduates of your school of nursing to raise funds for a student scholarship, you should be particularly creative so that all the graduates will read the opening, and the body, and the conclusion — and then send some money!

Try to visualize the individual to whom you are writing (audience) and even think about the setting in which he or she will be reading your letter (e.g., a busy office, with 17 other similar letters on the desk). Think about the information your reader will want, and try to present your message with consideration for the reader's point of view. What information does this person want or need in your letter?

The rules of the route for the business letter have been covered above. Adapt them to meet your needs (as source) as well as the needs of the message and the audience.

Finally, consider the tone of the letter. Try to see, again in your mind's eye, the recipient of your letter as a friend (even if you are writing a letter to complain about something). This visualization exercise will usually help you to set a good tone, and you can choose words that will make a positive impression. Is your business letter to be a begging letter, a demanding letter, a whining letter, a bitter letter? Even if the message is negative, you can use a positive tone; the reactions of your audience are likely to lead to better results. For example, if you are writing to complain about a mistake, the individual who gets the letter is probably not the one who made the mistake; why antagonize this person? If you get the reader on your side, the mistake is more likely to be corrected.

After thinking SMART, go over the steps of the writing PROCESS: Plan * Research * Organize * Create * Edit * Shine * Send! Just as with an assignment, if you take a few minutes to plan, research, and organize before you start to write your letter, you will write more like a pro. The letter is more likely to do what you want it to do. Of course, you should not spend hours or days on every simple letter. But the more important the letter, the more important it is to take time to plan, research, and organize so that the letter will be effective.

Think about letters of application for a job, for example. Suppose you write several letters quickly (without taking time to plan, research, organize, create, edit, and shine them before you submit them). You have wasted time and effort if those letters do not result in job interviews. Once you have done all the work for one letter, the next ones can almost be copied with only a little time needed to think SMART (e.g., Is this the same type of audience? Are the same skills required?). You may want to create a file of good letters that you can use as models. Many senior nurse managers do this.

Appendix C contains examples of letters that nurses might find helpful.

Keep your letter as short as possible. Businesspeople usually read one-page letters as soon as they open them; they put longer letters (especially those more than two pages) into the in-basket to read when they have more time (which is almost never!).

■ Memos

Memos are a vital part of a business environment, and if you are working in a hospital or other health care agency, you will likely have to write memos as part of your job. You therefore need to understand the rules of this route. Fortunately, many of the rules are similar to those for letters. In fact, memos are really just shorter, less formal letters done on a different type of stationery. For formal memos in some agencies, you may need to use all the parts of a business letter, including file numbers. On the other hand, some short handwritten memos are merely notes between two friends or colleagues confirming a time for lunch. Thinking SMART will help you.

The basic format for a memo is shown in Box 6.4. Note that the essential items in a memo are

- date;
- receiver's identity and department;
- sender's identity and departmental address and phone number;
- subject statement; and
- message (finishing with recommendations for follow-up).

The optional items in a memo include

- signature;
- copies (sometimes there is a section marked "Copies To:");
- enclosures or attachments;

- stenographic reference;
- file numbers; and
- security classification (in agencies where documents must be kept confidential).

Memo forms are often only 8.5" x 5.5", which should give you a clue about length. Keep your memos short, and usually keep them to one subject; it is often more efficient for your readers (always consider the audience) if you send two memos when you have two subjects. Doing so may not seem more convenient for you (source), but if the receiver can jot a short note in reply at the bottom of a memo and return it to you immediately, then you will get the action you want more quickly.

BOX 6.4 SAMPLE MEMO

Well Known Hospital
54321 Major Drive
Well Known City, BC   V4Z X0O

INTERDEPARTMENTAL MEMO

TO: *Mary Winters, Unit Manager OR*   DATE: *14/12/96*
FROM: *Glennis Zilm, Staff Library Volunteer*   PHONE: *555-1234*
SUBJECT: *Article on Latex Allergies*

You spoke to me some time ago about articles on latex allergies. Have you seen the following?

Latex Allergy Update: Clinical Practice and Unresolved Issues, by E. Meeropol. *WOCN: Journal of Wound, Ostomy and Continence Nursing*, Vol. 23, No. 4, July 1996.

This journal was recently donated to the library and has been placed on the "new reading" shelves. The article says those who have latex allergies often react as well when they eat certain foods, including bananas, avocados, and foods sterilized with ethylene oxide.

If you would like me to make a photocopy for you, please leave a message on my answering machine at home and I will do so the next time I am in the hospital.

Some agencies have supplies of "round trip memo forms," which allow you to write the original and one or two copies; they are used when you must keep a file related to that memo, such as might be required if you are sending a memo seeking action on a drug error or reporting a patient's fall. You keep the bottom copy for your records (e.g., perhaps attached to the patient's chart) and send the top copies. The receiver writes a reply for you at the bottom of the page, keeps the bottom copy for her or his files, and returns the original. These memos are often useful when you must send copies to keep others informed.

In some agencies, memos are intended to be posted on a bulletin board or filed in a binder so that all staff can see them. If so, you now have a new audience for your memo — and this readership should affect how you write the message. If the memo is to be posted, would it be more effective set up as a posterlike announcement? For example, if you are announcing the time and place of the unit's Christmas party, perhaps flyers on Christmas stationery prepared expressly for bulletin boards would be more effective than a memo. On the other hand, a poster would not be appropriate for a hospital policy directive that needs to reach all staff.

If the memo is to be filed in a binder on the unit, then you may want to consider how to make your memo more useful; for example, perhaps you should use 8.5" x 11" paper (rather than the shorter form) and ensure that holes are punched in the paper before it is sent. Sometimes it is more effective if the memo is circulated within a department rather than posted; if you believe that circulation would be the most efficient and make your message more useful, then you should attach a circulation list to the memo rather than expect the receiver to do that. Remember that each of the SMART elements interacts with and influences the others.

As you become more senior in your job, your attitude to and use of memos may change. Most staff nurses who attended my workshops reported that they resented memos, perhaps because many management memos seem to come across as "Now hear this" directives. Managers tend to write this way because they have a responsibility to communicate, and "Do this" memos usually seem quick and effective. When you join the management team, however, you can take action to reduce the negative impact that this type of memo seems to have on staff. For example, when you become a head nurse or unit manager, you can try to send fewer memos and have more face-to-face meetings with staff. You can set up headline cards (e.g., "New Directives From

Pharmacy") and then post all policy memos from pharmacy in that section of the bulletin board. Or you may choose to file them in special binders in which staff can review them. You can review incoming memos yourself and use a highlighter to emphasize relevant points for your staff. These hints, however, relate more to management techniques than to writing skills.

The important point is to think SMART when it comes to writing memos. If you make them short, simple, clear, interesting, friendly, appropriate, and easy for the receiver to handle, your memos will be effective.

■ E-Mail

Within many hospitals and agencies, e-mail messages and other forms of electronic communication (e.g., scheduling of meetings) have replaced many of the telephone calls and the short, informal memos that were so common in the past. E-mail messages are a special form of written communication, and the SMART elements apply. Possibly, you already use e-mail to communicate with friends, but these messages are likely informal. E-mail used for business messages will take on a slightly more formal tone. Generally, e-mail messages can be viewed as shorter, quicker, slightly less formal memos. Once again, the tone can range from strictly formal (using a memo format and formal language) to highly informal — perhaps with contractions and even added "smilies" such as :)!

Usually, e-mail messages are short and to the point. Within agencies, e-mail is used because it is quicker than interdepartmental mail and less intrusive than telephone calls. Between agencies, it is often used because it is cheaper than long distance phone calls and much faster than regular post office delivery ("snail mail"). If a message is longer than can easily be read on a single screen, the receiver will have to scroll through the message, although he or she may elect to print it out. Either is more time consuming, so keep your e-mail messages short. The format for e-mail documents is often determined by the software programs used or by the telecommunications system that supplies the on-line service.

If you use a computer often, you will no doubt be familiar with the emotional conversational styles (tone) that can be conveyed through typing. For example, use of all CAPITAL LETTERS is generally considered "shouting." You will often see typing errors and many of the common errors in informal e-mail messages — but why waste time and energy if the point of your message is to ask someone if she is ready to go for lunch?

Use the SMART principles. Is the e-mail route suitable for your message? Do you need to transfer printed information quickly? Does the format matter? The basic e-mail format is usually best suited for short messages, although if you know how you can attach files and send a document. For example, you can send an assignment or a report via e-mail as an attached file, which can then be printed by the receiver. This method works wonderfully for the exchange of draft documents, but often the formatting is not suitable for finished documents. You also need to consider whether your receiver likes to use e-mail and file transfer — and whether he or she knows how.

■ Résumés

One of the important written communications you will need during your nursing career is a résumé. A résumé (sometimes written without the accents) is a brief summary of educational and employment experiences that is submitted with a job application. In today's world, chances are that you will change jobs during your working lifetime *at least* six times; for many nurses, up to 15 different jobs during their working careers is common. Sometimes these changes are within a single agency, but sometimes you may even decide to change to a different field.

To develop a good résumé and keep it up to date so that you can apply for positions in coming years, consider starting a résumé file for yourself. In it, you can keep all the important background materials that you will need in future years, such as your high school certificate, nursing graduation certificates, registration examination results, copies of official documents pertaining to courses and marks, and information on special courses taken (e.g., CPR certificate). These documents will come in handy for many years and will help you to keep dates correct. (Believe me, you will forget such information!) Start a good file, and keep copies of your résumés in it for future reference.

A résumé may not be so important for that first nursing job after graduation, but it will become more and more important in later years. Hospitals and most other health care agencies generally prefer that applicants for staff nurse positions fill out an application form designed especially for them; it makes it easy for a personnel officer to review the information quickly and according to the special needs of the hospital or agency. If that is the case, you must fill out the form — but you can also attach your résumé, which carries additional weight and shows that you know something about job hunting. Furthermore, if you have your résumé on hand when you fill out the application form, you are more likely to have all the information (e.g., dates) you need. So you should develop a résumé, or at least a worksheet that you can follow when filling out applications, soon after graduation.

You can hire other people to help you prepare and type a résumé, but if you learn how to do it yourself, by thinking SMART, you will end up with a much better message. Unless you have good computer skills, you may need to hire a typist, but the most useful résumé tends to be the one you have prepared yourself.

A résumé is usually your first contact with a potential employer, so, most importantly, you need to weigh the needs of the receiver. Most employers spend less than a minute looking over a résumé when it first arrives, so consider using ways to make yours stand out in a pile of other résumés. You could have it printed in fancy type on shocking pink paper with a color copy of your photo at the top — but does such a résumé convey the non-verbal message you want to send? Such a résumé might be useful if you are applying to an ad agency or talent bureau, but most health care employers expect a more professional approach from nurses. For most health care employers, your résumé should be short, clear, well organized, and neat so that the essential points can be assessed quickly.

You need to consider some important things about yourself as a source. When you are looking for your first job in a tight job market, you may need to send out several résumés at once. If your budget is slim, you may wish to develop one general résumé that can be photo-copied and used for several potential employers, such as several hospitals in an urban area. Or, if you can use a computer, you may wish to develop a good general format, but adapt each résumé to fit the needs of each potential employer, such as a pediatric ward, a home care agency, or a geriatric facility.

A résumé alone will not get you a job. The purpose of a résumé is to get you a job interview. Potential employers develop a short list of possible employees based on their résumés (or application forms), so you should know how to develop a good one. Because a potential employer will generally spend less than a minute glancing over the résumé, you need to supply all the important information in one or two pages.

CONTENT FOR A RÉSUMÉ

Most résumés fall into one of two broad categories: chronological and functional. The chronological résumé is the most common and concentrates on supplying details about your educational and employment history. The functional résumé allows you to tell more about the various jobs you have held. You need to keep information suitable for both types in your résumé file because this material will be useful when you fill out applications for nursing positions and when you go to interviews. However, the basic content is similar for both and includes the following categories. Sample résumés are shown in Boxes 6.5 and 6.6.

Name, address, and phone number

They should be given clearly at the top of the first page. You do not usually supply other personal information (e.g., marital status, family, age, weight, height, and so on) in the résumé, and never at the top.

Education

List the highlights of your education in chronological order, starting with the most recent educational preparation and working back. When you graduate and are applying for your first positions, you may want to include your high school graduation, although employers will generally assume that, if you have graduated from a college or university, then you have completed high school. As you determine whether to include high school graduation, think SMART: source (are you young, inexperienced, and applying for a first position, or are you older, experienced, and applying for a senior position?); message (is your educational experience or your work experience more important to this potential employer?); audience (would this information be relevant to this reader?); route (have I room to include all the details?); and tone (is this a full-length, formal application in which I should include all relevant information?).

Information about relevant non-credit education may also be included in this section, such as information about short courses (e.g., CPR courses, or courses in operating room or neonatal care). You would definitely include information on certificate courses.

BOX 6.5 *Sample Chronological Résumé (New Graduate)*

Résumé
NOEL KANE, R.N.
Apt. 12 — 1812 Bayview Street
Surrey, B.C. V4B 0X0
Telephone: (604) 555-3238

Job Objective: Registered Nurse Staff Position, Surrey District Hospital

Education:

1997 Registered Nurse Degree
School of Nursing
Chinook Community College
Sardis, B.C.

1994 High School Graduation (with honors)
Duke of Connaught Senior Secondary
South Surrey, B.C.

Work Background:

1996 (Feb.) - 1997 (June) Kitchen Assistant (weekend relief)
Sardis Memorial Hospital, Sardis, B.C.

1994 (June-July) Kitchen Assistant
Sardis Memorial Hospital, Sardis, B.C.

Awards:

1994 University Women's Club (South Fraser Branch) Ethel
Singh Scholarship ($1,000 for further study)

Professional Memberships:

1997 - Registered Nurses Association of B.C.

1995 - 1997 Canadian Student Nurses Association (national
vice-president, 1996-97)

References:
Mr. J. R. Toews R.R.3, Box 17, Sardis, B.C. V6M 0X1
(604) 555-2198

Mrs. Cheryl Jones School of Nursing, Chinook Community
College, Sardis, B.C. V7K 1X0
(604) 555-2176, local 546

(Prepared August 1997)

BOX 6.6 *Sample Functional Résumé (Recent Graduate)*

Résumé

MARTHA CHUNG, RN, BSN

#91 — 2488 Johnston Road
Edmonton, AB   T6G 0X0
Telephone: (403) 555-3723

Job Objective: Unit Manager, Post-Anesthetic Recovery Unit, Edmonton General

Work Background:

1996 (June) - present Staff Nurse PAR Unit Edmonton General	RN staff duties in 18-bed PAR Responsible for orientation of new staff Developed CPR Cart for Emergency Unit and for Main Building
1995 (Aug.) - 1996 (May) Staff Nurse Emergency Department Queenston General Queenston, ON	RN staff duties in a 24-bed, 24- hour Emergency Unit During last six months worked per- manent night (1900 - 0700 hours) and was senior nurse-in-charge

Education:

1995 (June)   CPR Certification Course, Boston University Hospital, Boston
(five-week specialty course)

1995   Bachelor of Science in Nursing (with honors)
Faculty of Nursing
King's University
Queenston, ON

Professional Memberships:
Alberta Association of Registered Nurses
College of Nurses of Ontario

Publications:
Chow, E. K., & Chung, M. (1996). Safety precautions for crash cart medications. *RN Communiqué, 4*(3), 6-7.

Personal Information:
Age 28 years, married with one child
Fluent in Cantonese
Hobbies: five-pin bowling, swimming (Red Cross Life Saving Certificate)

References:
Available on request

(Prepared August 1997)

Work experience

This section of your résumé will change most throughout your career. At first, you will not have much to include here, but you should regularly update your résumé files even if you do not need to develop a new résumé for each job.

If you are early in your career, you may wish to include information on part-time work even if it does not seem relevant to the job for which you are applying. One personnel officer told me that when he is reviewing for junior positions, he notes whether the applicant has worked summers at fast-food outlets such as McDonald's or A&W; he said that individuals who have managed to hold those jobs probably have a good overall work ethic. Sometimes volunteer work should be mentioned in this section as well; for example, if you worked every Thursday after classes throughout high school as a "Candy Stripper" volunteer feeding patients in a geriatric ward of the hospital to which you are applying, you should include this information.

When you are further along in your career, you would list your various positions in chronological order, working back from the most recent. You could separate positions to mark advancements even though these positions were for the same employer, such as:

1996 - present	Unit Manager, Surgical Ward, Peace Arch Hospital, White Rock
1994 - 1996 (Aug.)	Staff Nurse, Surgical Ward, Peace Arch Hospital, White Rock

Later in your career, when you need to list several positions, you might combine these two.

Honors

In this section, which should be brief and to the point, you can include scholarships and awards.

Professional memberships

You need to include information on your nursing registration and to indicate in which province(s) you are registered. If you are hired, you will need to provide your registration number, but as this is an important and confidential number I suggest that you do not put it on the résumé. Because provincial registration implies membership in the

Canadian Nurses Association, you can decide whether to mention this membership or not. You should include all current professional memberships, and you may elect to include some or all past professional memberships. For example, if you held office in a professional nursing association in another province but are no longer a member, this information may still be relevant because it indicates involvement in professional activities. You would not usually include membership in civic, church, or social groups unless you believe that they are relevant to your audience and your message.

Publications

In this section, you list all your professional publications. Early in your career, you may not have many. If you eventually go into nursing education, the list of publications will likely be much longer. You must not trim this section in later years; a list of publications should be complete and uncensored — even if an article eventually seems immature or unimportant. In later years, you may wish to put a lengthy publication list on separate sheets and attach them only when relevant.

Personal information

This section creates controversy. You are not required to give information such as age, marital status, or number of children, but sometimes this information is relevant (see example of the functional résumé). For example, if you are seeking a daytime job because you have a child and wish to be home in the evenings, you may want to make this point on your résumé (and in your covering letter). Many people believe that information about hobbies should never be included on a résumé — and that is appropriate for them as sources! Sometimes, however, information about extracurricular activities gives a potential employer an idea of the person behind the facts. Obviously, you have to think SMART and make up your own mind.

References

The inclusion of references with a résumé is another controversial point. Some agencies require that you supply them; others prefer to get in touch with one or more of your previous employers directly. It is certainly appropriate to say "References available on request," or you can simply omit this section. If you do use names, you should first ask the individuals if they are willing to give you a good recommendation.

Date

All résumés should be dated at the bottom of the page to ensure that an old one is not considered current. You need not sign the résumé.

POINTS TO REMEMBER ABOUT RÉSUMÉS

- Be accurate and truthful. Some prospective employers check the information. Furthermore, your résumé may form part of your permanent work record. Do not exaggerate responsibilities or try to oversell yourself!
- Be as brief as possible. One page is good; two full pages are maximum (even for senior administrators). Applicants for teaching positions at universities may use longer résumés.
- Double-check grammar, spelling, and punctuation. Use action words (e.g., developed, co-ordinated, supervised) when possible. Use point form or short paragraphs and the same verb tense throughout.
- Pay attention to visual presentation. A résumé should never look cramped — and should never be soiled or messy.
- Use a covering letter (see Appendix C).
- Never underestimate yourself. A résumé is an advertisement for you; it is intended to get you an interview.

■ Reports

Reports are another standard way to send a message. They require the same SMART thinking and follow the same PROCESS as other written communications. The message, of course, could be delivered in many formats, but the report route is used when the message is longer and requires more detailed background than in a memo or letter. The tone tends to be more formal, although a report can range from slightly informal (between two colleagues working on a project) to highly formal (a royal commission report to a federal or provincial government). The audience can vary from a single individual to the general public, although reports tend to be shared with larger groups, so there is a primary audience (the individual or small group who requested the report) and a secondary audience (the larger group with whom the primary audience may share the report). For a royal commission report, the individual to whom the report is addressed in the covering letter may be the prime minister, but if the report is approved and released by the government, it may appear as a publication for the Canadian public. An annual report from a unit manager to the vice-president of nursing may end up being shared with the executive committee, the financial department, and the president of the hospital auxiliary, and even reproduced in the hospital's annual report to the public. Hence, a good starting point for an individual asked to prepare a report is to find out exactly who needs the report and what its purpose is to be.

In other words, if you are asked to prepare a report, you need to follow the writing PROCESS — especially the first three steps before you go any higher on the ladder. As part of your research, get copies of previous reports that may help you to understand the particular format used for that kind of report in your agency, but get other kinds of reports as well so that you can make innovative and creative changes. Obviously, if you are a hospital unit manager preparing a quarterly report, you will keep it simpler in format and layout than if you are an advertising agency manager preparing an annual report for the shareholders of Canada's largest bank.

Remember, however, that the message continues to be the point of a written communication. Be certain that you understand the message and what its purpose is for its audience. Are you asked to provide a report with data on various brands of infant cots so that a committee of several head nurses can make a decision? Or are you asked to recommend the brand of infant cots that should be purchased based on *your* research and expertise? In the former, you will need to provide all the background details on the various infant cots available, including costs, safety factors, ease of use, and other such details, so that the committee can debate the issue and make an informed decision; the purpose of the research report is to save the committee time. In the latter, you can be much more direct and brief and state that, based on your research and testing and after consideration of prices, you (an expert source) recommend the "Babe Cot" as the most suitable of six cots currently on the market. You might choose to support your recommendation briefly in the report and to include appendices that give background information on all the cots, but the main body of the report should be brief, to the point, and based on your expertise, because the purpose of your report is to *recommend*. In the latter instance, the committee might simply approve your report and send it on to the purchasing department — so you should include all the details the matériels manager will need to go ahead and make the order.

For reports in which you are asked to give an opinion or recommendation, you can use the acronym PRESS:

Position: state your position clearly.
Reason: state the reason you are for or against.
Example: give an example or two to illustrate your position.
Support: support your position with statistics and facts.
Summarize: close with a brief summary of your position.

Some reports fall halfway between the informational report and the recommendation report; these are termed interpretive reports, which not only inform and describe but also analyze. The interpretive report, however, does not usually make recommendations. Progress reports fall into this category.

Proposals, including grant proposals and project requests, also come under the category of reports. Important sections of these reports include proposed costs (budget) and methods of implementation; a time schedule is also useful. If you are applying for a grant from a foundation, each one usually has specific forms that are used; check with the foundation before starting work (i.e., during the planning step of the PROCESS ladder). As part of planning, you may also want to borrow (or, if report writing is going to be a major part of your job, even buy) a book on how to write reports. Yes, there are books on how to write reports and even on how to write certain kinds of reports (e.g., writing proposals, or writing technical reports). This section provides only an overview of reports. You should also review Appendix D to find recommended books on reports.

FORMAT OF A REPORT

A good report follows the traditional outline described in detail earlier in this book. The essentials are introduction, body, and conclusion. There is one slight difference, however. In most written communications, the introduction merely "Tells them what you are going to tell them" — and it does so in broad terms. In a report, the introduction *summarizes* what you are going to tell your audience and is specific about conclusions, recommendations, and actions to be taken. In other words, you give the essence of the report on the first page.

You provide a summary at the beginning because of the audience. For many readers of a business report, the summary is all that is required. If the reader needs more details, he or she can go deeper into the report — but most readers do not want to read the whole report to discover "the bottom line." Furthermore, the organization of the body of the report is based on this premise: you make it easy, through the organization, for a reader to find the details he or she needs.

If you hand out reports during a meeting, and the chair allows the members time to look at the report, observe how they react. Typically, about 80% of committee members will turn quickly to page 1 and start to read. If the opening on page 1 catches their interest with some solid information, they will continue to read all of page 1 and turn to page 2. About 40% of typical committee members continue to read page 2 (provided that the message stays relevant); the other 60% let their attention wander and may even start flipping through the rest of the report (many will turn to the end to look for conclusions there) or turn to other committee matters. Only about 10% will continue to read on to page 3. The same pattern is followed when individuals get your report in their offices; about 80% of them turn immediately to page 1. Depending on their time and the importance of the report to them, they will stay with it for page 2 and maybe page 3 — and then set the report aside to read when they have more time (which, for most busy people, is never). Thus, where should you put the important message in your report?

In the 1970s, reports typically started with all the background, went through the history of why the report was needed, and built to the conclusion on the last few pages. More recent reports start with conclusions and recommendations, followed by the reasons for the recommendations, and the background and historical perspective (if included at all) tend to be near the end. The former style is still used occasionally, usually for expository or traditional reports; the latter style is considered motivational and is more likely to be used in hospitals and health care agencies.

The standard organization for a detailed report would thus follow this route (you will probably notice similarities to the student assignments described earlier in this book):

- **cover** (if necessary), with a good, catchy title;
- **title page(s)**, including information on authors or compilers, place, date, and other relevant material;
- **preliminary pages**, including table of contents (and perhaps a list of tables, graphs, or illustrations if used) if the report is more than 20 pages; in major reports, you may also need a preface and acknowledgments (but keep them brief);

- **introduction** — frequently entitled "Executive Summary" — in which the report is summarized in one or at most two pages; the introduction may even be put before the preliminary pages to make it stand out;
- **body of report**, which includes some or all of these elements:
  - synopsis or abstract of the body;
  - background (the why of this report);
  - method used to look into the subject (how you did it);
  - findings (with *all* the facts, including financial information);
  - discussion (including your interpretation of the facts, your recommendations in detail, and your conclusions in detail);
  - concluding section of the body (which ties the whole report together and reiterates the executive summary);
- **references and bibliography**; and
- **appendices** (*after* references and bibliography because usually they are attachments that you did not write).

Not all reports will follow this format, of course; it depends on Source * Message * Audience * Route * Tone. For example, some hospital administrations require quarterly and annual reports from department heads and have strict rules about format. One hospital vice-president asked her department heads to organize their quarterly reports this way:

1. Brief introductory statement followed by sections on progress since the last report (were goals met?)
2. Body giving statements and comparison figures on
   2.1 budget
   2.2 staffing
   2.3 administrative problems
   2.4 in-service education activities
   2.5 committee participation
   2.6 other relevant activities
3. Concluding section that includes a list of new long-term and short-term goals.

This vice-president also wanted her department heads to use a modified Harvard numbering style whereby each section in the body of the report used her specific numbering system and each paragraph in each section had a number. Thus, the first paragraph in the budget section was 2.1.1, the second paragraph was numbered 2.1.2, and so on. The department heads knew exactly what was expected by this particular audience and could prepare their reports accordingly.

SHORT REPORTS ("BRIEFS")

The term "brief" has come into business use during the 1990s. Generally speaking, a brief is a *short* report usually recommending some kind of action or some solution to a problem. The term has been around much longer in the legal profession, in which a brief is a concise statement intended to inform other, usually more senior, counsellors about a client's case. No doubt you have also heard the term used in military circles in the form "briefing." The idea is to get a summary of a lot of information into a short, usable form for someone who knows less about a subject than you do but who is in a position to take action.

Professional associations often present briefs to political committees or commissions. A written brief or short report is taken to the committee's meeting, and a representative of the association gives an even briefer oral presentation and answers questions (e.g., to a royal commission on health care and costs). In these instances, a brief is a longer and more formal document than a letter or memo; a brief might contain 750 to 1,000 words (three to five pages), which would be a l-o-n-g letter!

The shortest reports can be sent as memos. For example, if a senior nurse administrator in your hospital asks you for a report on the status of a grant given to your department by the hospital auxiliary, he or she probably does not want a formal layout. An example of a short progress report sent as a memo is given in Appendix C.

HELPFUL HINTS ABOUT REPORTS

- Keep your report as short as possible — the briefer the better.
- Summarize your message on page 1.
- Keep the body of your report as brief as possible; use tables to summarize and present information visually; put background details into appendices.
- Keep the purpose of the report in mind — is it to inform, persuade, request, analyze, or recommend?
- Do you want the receivers of the report to take action? If so, be specific about the action you want them to take, and request it on page 1.
- Recommend solutions if you identify problems.
- Provide full information related to cost if relevant; in today's world, report readers are concerned about budgets.

■ Research Papers and Theses

If you are in the final years of a baccalaureate nursing degree program or in a program for your master's degree, you may be asked to prepare a research paper, which represents another specialized route with many rules. The fourth edition of the *Publication Manual of the American Psychological Association* (APA, 1994) provides an overview. Two other excellent resources are *How to Write and Publish a Scientific Paper* (fourth edition), by Robert A. Day (1993), and *Scientific Writing for Graduate Students*, published by the Council of Biology Editors (1986). Other resources are identified in Appendix D.

As a route, a research paper (sometimes called a research report) follows many of the rules already described in this book for student assignments and reports. Sometimes a thesis is actually a research report. To prepare a research report, as with all written communications, you need to implement the SMART essentials and follow the writing PROCESS.

A research paper reports on the findings of a research project; usually, the writer is the principal researcher or a member of the research team that planned and carried out the project. By the time you are asked to prepare a research paper, you will have read numerous research reports and articles, and you will have taken or will be taking a course on the development of a research project.

Most likely, the project itself will start with the development of a research question or problem. Students often agonize over the evolution of a good research question. An excellent place to find one is in a nursing setting; ask staff nurses what problems they find in their day-to-day work, and then pose those problems as a research question. The preparation of the research question itself is a major task; if you do a good job of it, you will find it much easier later to write the research article or report. Follow the SMART approach and go through the steps of the writing PROCESS. It is crucial that you do research on the question itself before you commit yourself to a project. Eventually, you will write an abstract summarizing the research question and get it approved before you begin the project. You may also need to write a funding proposal related to the research project. Once you start looking into background material for the project, you will write up a literature review. Once you have done the review, you will need to identify the method that you are going to use in the written communication. Every step of the research process involves a new written communication. You may actually write up many of the stages as you proceed through the project. Once you have carried out the research, you are ready to prepare the final report.

FORMAT OF A RESEARCH PAPER

Most research reports follow the traditional, rigid scientific method of organization, which has become known as IMRAD, an acronym for Introduction, Method, Results, and Discussion. It follows the same format, with a few variations, as that already described for reports and student assignments. Many of the variations depend on the audience — the instructor for your course or the supervisor of your thesis committee. However, in general, the following show a basic format for a research paper, although the order of items will depend on the expectations of your audience:

- **title page** — usually has some rigid rules: it is longer and more formal in tone, and it accurately describes the contents of the paper so that it can be retrieved easily in a literature search; usually, there is no cover for a research paper, so the title page includes name(s) and title(s) of author(s) or project team, as well as address, date, and other relevant material;
- **preliminary pages**, including the table of contents, a list of tables, graphs, or illustrations, and perhaps a preface and acknowledgments;
- **abstract** — which is written last and which summarizes the project and report, although it may or may not give details of the findings (depending on the interpretation of your instructor); there may be a restriction on the length of the abstract (e.g., 125 words maximum, or one page maximum), and an abstract rarely takes more than two pages;
- **body of research paper**, which includes some or all of these elements:
  - introduction (which may be labelled as such in a research paper; includes history of or background to the project);
  - statement of research question/hypothesis/objectives of the study;
  - literature review;
  - research method(s) used (may include subsections on design, sample, data collection, and methods for analyzing data);
  - statement on human rights protection or other approvals needed;
  - statement on limitations of the study (may be positioned after results or as a subsection under the conclusion);

- results/findings (what you found out, with *all* the facts, including all statistical data);
- discussion/interpretation (your analysis of and comment on the facts in detail; may require subsections in a long study);
- conclusions (if the project reached any; they may be included under the discussion section);
- recommendations/applications (if the project reached any; may be included under the discussion section or under the conclusion section);
- concluding section for the body of the research report (may be omitted if you let the conclusions and recommendations themselves end and round out the paper); and
- appendices (in a research paper or thesis, they come before the references and bibliography because usually you prepare any appendices);
- **references and bibliography; and**
- **index** (may be required, although this is a new idea).

HELPFUL HINTS FOR RESEARCH PAPERS/THESES

- If this is a student project, discuss *everything* with your instructor (or thesis committee) as early as possible in the project and regularly as you proceed.
- Preparation of these papers is usually a massive project, so break it down into small stages, with deadlines, and never leave it until the last minute.

■ Articles

At some time in your nursing career, you may want to write an article for a professional journal; nurses often want to share good ideas with other nurses. The basic SMART elements and the writing PROCESS will also help you to prepare a good article that has a chance of being accepted by the editor and published in the journal.

As you contemplate the SMART elements, carefully consider yourself as a source. Can you speak authoritatively? Would someone be interested in your views on the subject? You can write an article as a student as long as you provide a student's viewpoint or interpretation. If you have spent a year or more researching a specific topic and gathering data that are new and pertinent, then you can write as a researcher. If you are elected as an officer of an association, you may be able to write on behalf of the members of that association. Just be sure that you recognize your role in writing the article.

The route will be a certain journal, so you need to be familiar with that journal. Look at its guidelines and format to see whether your message will be appropriate. Once you really look at professional journals as a possible author, you will discover that there are many different kinds (e.g., research journals, general interest journals, specialty journals, newsletters, abstract journals) and that within any one journal there are often different kinds of articles (e.g., news items, letters to the editor, editorials, opinion articles, general articles, research articles, book reviews). In the early 1990s, more than 100 professional journals were published specifically for nurses, and nearly 300 other professional journals in related fields accepted articles from nurses. Which journal and which type of article would be best suited to your message? To see the range of professional journals, visit the journals section of a large biomedical library. The library in your professional nurses' association headquarters usually carries a wide range of nursing journals, and the librarian there can provide you with a list of current nursing journals.

You also need to consider the readership of the journal, which will eventually make up your audience. If your message is directed to physicians, it will not be accepted if you send it to a nursing journal; for example, *The Canadian Nurse* is not likely to accept an article telling doctors that they need to write more legibly. Some journals are directed to all registered nurses in a particular region (e.g., *The Canadian Nurse*, or the journal published by a provincial nurses' association or union). Others have special audiences, such as nursing administrators (e.g., *The Canadian Journal of Nursing Administration*) or those interested in nursing research (e.g., *The Canadian Journal of Nursing Research/Revue canadienne de recherche en sciences infirmières*).

You can often gain a good understanding of the readers of the journal by reading the information, usually in small print, on the masthead. The masthead will also give you other information, such as the names of the editors, the address of the journal, its frequency of publication, its cost and whether it is sold by subscription or sent only to members, and, usually, whether it welcomes unsolicited manuscripts for review. Sometimes the masthead will tell you the number of copies that are printed for circulation and that you should write to the editors for guidelines and information before you submit an article.

As well, if you look through several issues of the journal, you will find that editors publish a page containing "Information for Authors" and sometimes a "Call for Papers" asking for articles related to specific topics. As a potential author, you should make careful note of these pages. (They may not be included in every issue, but they usually appear at least once a year.) The Information for Authors advises you about length and rules of the route and usually mentions which style guide should be followed.

You will also learn a great deal about the route and the audience simply by reviewing several copies of the journal for which you want to write. When you first begin to write articles for professional journals, it is a good idea to submit to a journal that you read regularly. If you review all the issues for the past year, you will get a good idea of recent topics and whether the tone is formal (as in most research journals) or slightly less formal (as in the journals for a general nursing audience, such as *The Canadian Nurse* or *Nursing 98*). You could note whether the journal tends to use short, catchy titles or longer, research-oriented titles. You could see whether each article opens with an abstract. You could determine the messages that get published. You could notice the length of most articles (and even estimate the number of words on a page to give you an idea of length). You could check whether the journal uses photographs or not. All these points will affect how you eventually approach your message.

Most articles fall into one of these categories:

- research articles, which are similar to, but often shorter than, research reports;
- informational articles on procedures, processes, and techniques (often called "how to" articles);
- case studies, which describe in detail the care of a patient (either a typical or an unusual case); these reports used to be common in nursing journals but have been published less frequently in recent years;
- historical articles, which may or may not follow a special historical research format;
- articles on current issues, which are often called "opinion pieces" but which include some in-depth analysis of the various views on a new or controversial matter; and
- editorials, which are usually solicited by the staff of the journal.

QUERY LETTER

Before you spend too much time creating a manuscript, you should, as part of the steps plan, research, and organize, ask the editor of the journal about possible interest in your subject. Once you have determined the topic, you can send what is known as a "query letter" to the editor(s) of the journal(s) that you believe would best convey your message to the appropriate readers. A sample query letter is given in Appendix C. You can send more than one query letter at a time to see which journal(s) would be interested in your article. On the other hand, you *never* send a finished manuscript to more than one journal at a time.

You can send a query letter when you are at the outline step in the writing PROCESS; the reply will help you to create an appropriate first draft and to use the right style guide for the final draft. You will not want to proceed to later steps if the editor replies that the journal has already accepted an article on the topic you suggested and is only interested in reviewing your article if you focus on some specific aspect of the broader subject.

When you first begin to write for publication, you should work out a detailed outline for your article before you send out query letters; in other words, you need to know what your message is going to be so that you can describe it briefly for an editor. You also need to provide enough information about yourself (and your co-authors, if any) so that the editor can judge whether you are a good source for the proposed topic. Your query letter will also be stronger and more impressive to an editor if you indicate that you are familiar with the journal and its contents and know something about its readers (e.g., whether it is a specialty journal directed mainly to pediatric nurses working in Britain).

FORMAT FOR AN ARTICLE

The format for an article depends on the type of message, the requirements of the journal, and the potential readers. Usually, when an editor replies to your query letter, he or she encloses information about the format expected. As well, you will know from an examination of the previous issues just what kind of format is expected.

In general, the format for an article will follow those described earlier for student assignments, reports, and research papers. A few sections are omitted, and additional items may be required. The following is a general guide:

- **covering letter** (see Appendix C);
- **title page** — includes name(s) and title(s) of author(s), address and phone numbers of one author (usually the principal author, listed first in the by-line) who will be the main contact, and date submitted;
- **abstract** (if asked for by the journal) — usually provided on a separate sheet, but check the style requirements;
- **text of manuscript**, including the title at the top of the first page and subheadings as required; authors' names and identifying information should not be given in the text, only on the title page, so that the article may be sent out for "blind review" by peers; organization should be similar to that for a short general article, but if the article is to be published in a research journal, the headings should follow the IMRAD layout recommended for research reports;
- **tables or figures** (and, occasionally, photographs or other artwork; check with the editor before sending photographs and artwork); and
- **references** — check the style used in the journal; some journals keep references to an absolute minimum, whereas others allow long lists of references; there is usually no bibliography.

Note that journals usually require several copies of the complete manuscript (including the title page). Check the Information for Authors sheet and send photocopies as required. You do not need to supply extra copies of the covering letter.

The following items may also be required by the journal and will be asked for in the response to your query letter:

- **copyright transmittal sheet**, signed by all authors, supplied by the journal or described in detail in the Information for Authors sheet;
- **sheet with "callouts"** (some journals call them "pull quotes"), which are short quotations selected from the article and highlighted on the cover or in the page layout to catch reader interest (some editors ask authors to supply them);
- **computer disk**, clearly marked with your name, the title of the article, and the hardware and software used (e.g., MS-DOS, WordPerfect for Windows 6.1); you may also include a typed list of the files on the disk with a brief description (e.g., TAB1 — Table 1, produced using Windows Graphics);
- **permission forms for use of copyrighted material** (including photographs by a professional photographer); for more information about these forms, consult the style manual recommended by the journal or ask the editor what is required; and

- **permission forms for subjects in photographs** (if you have taken photographs to use with your article, you need to supply permissions from individuals shown in the photographs to protect patients/clients).

Copyright is a complicated subject. You automatically hold the copyright for original material that you produce as soon as it is written down. Almost all professional journals require that you transfer to them copyright *for the specific material that they publish*. This copyright gives a journal control of the material once it is published; anyone who wishes to reproduce or use significant portions of your work thus needs to obtain permission from the journal editors (not from you). This also means that if you wish to reproduce the material (e.g., to use it later in a book), you also must obtain permission from the journal that originally published it. Although this may seem unfair, it is common practice with scientific and professional journals. Some well-known writers are able to work out special arrangements with journal editors and transfer to the journal only "first serial rights"; this method is frequently used by novelists, short story writers, and poets. Limited transmittals can become complicated, however; anyone who wishes to reproduce your work after several years may have difficulty finding you (whereas he or she could almost always locate the journal's address). By assigning copyright for your article to a journal, you make it easy both to share your scientific/professional work and to control its reproduction. If you do not sign a copyright transmittal sheet, many journals will not even accept your manuscript for review. (The copyright transfer also helps the journal to protect your manuscript from unlawful use by reviewers.) As I said, copyright is complicated; some lawyers make it their special field. If you have questions or concerns, refer to a book on copyright matters or discuss the point with the editor of the journal — or with your lawyer.

HELPFUL HINT FOR ARTICLES

- The briefer the better: short articles stand a much better chance of being accepted for publication than do long ones.

■ Summary

Throughout your career as a nurse, you will need to prepare hundreds of written communications. Furthermore, the styles and formats of these written communications will likely change many times during your lifetime, largely because of changes in technology. For example, the layout of business letters has changed markedly during the last century; the first changes occurred when businesses switched from handwritten to typed letters. In the last 25 years, letter-writing styles have changed several times, largely because of the introduction of computers.

Because of computers, moreover, footnotes in essays could come back into fashion and replace the author-year style. In the future, students may need to know how to submit their assignments to their instructors electronically (e.g., on disk or by file transfer through e-mail). Computer software will likely improve so that margins are set and reset automatically. Already some nursing courses are offered over the Internet and all communication is electronic.

The format of reports will change because much information formerly compiled and kept by individual departments (e.g., staffing figures, patient census) will be available to qualified personnel through the agency's computer system. Submission of articles to journals will change as well. More and more on-line journals will appear, and they will likely accept manuscript submissions from authors through file transfer.

So, although the formats described in these chapters will be useful to you, the most important things to learn from the book are the application of the SMART elements of communication and the use of the writing PROCESS. Their principles will last for your lifetime. Once you have learned how to use these principles, you are on the road to growth as a writer, no matter how styles change.

■ References

American Psychological Association. (1994). *Publication manual of the American Psychological Association* (4th ed.). Washington, DC: Author.

Council of Biology Editors. (1986). *Scientific writing for graduate students: A manual on the teaching of scientific writing.* Bethesda, MD: Author.

Day, R. A. (1993). *How to write and publish a scientific paper* (4th ed.). Phoenix: Oryx Press.

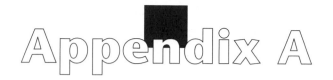

Appendix A

Examples of APA Style for Full Citations in Reference Lists and Bibliographies

The following examples of APA style illustrate the most common forms that first-year nursing students would require for formal papers. Note that sometimes you need to combine elements from one example with another (e.g., group as author, illustrated in a book example, for a journal article). For more details and examples, please consult the *Publication Manual of the American Psychological Association*, fourth edition, prepared and published in 1994 by the American Psychological Association, Washington, DC.

BOOK, SINGLE AUTHOR

Buckley, J. (1995). <u>Fit to print: The Canadian student's guide to essay writing.</u> Toronto: Harcourt Brace Canada.

In body of paper: (Buckley, 1995); with a quotation: (Buckley, 1995, p. xx).

Points to notice: position of period in relation to parentheses; capitals are used only for first letters in each section of the title of a book and for proper nouns (note differences for journals below); the apostrophe in "student's" — be certain you have copied it correctly.

BOOK, TWO AUTHORS

Zilm, G., & Warbinek, E. (1994). <u>Legacy: History of nursing education at the University of British Columbia 1919-1994.</u> Vancouver: University of British Columbia School of Nursing.

In body of paper: (Zilm & Warbinek, 1994); with a quotation: (Zilm & Warbinek, 1994, p. xx).

Point to notice: use of commas around authors' initials.

BOOK, TWO EDITORS

Hibberd, J. M., & Kyle, M. E. (Eds.). (1994). <u>Nursing management in Canada.</u> Toronto: Saunders.

In body of paper: (Hibberd & Kyle, 1994); with a quotation: (Hibberd & Kyle, 1994, p. xx).

Point to notice: the period both inside and after the parentheses for "Eds."

BOOK, TWO EDITORS, SECOND EDITION

Baumgart, A. J., & Larsen, J. (Eds.). (1992). <u>Canadian nursing faces the future</u> (2nd ed.). Toronto: Mosby-Year Book.

In body of paper: you probably would not refer to such material in the body of the paper because each chapter was written by different authors, and you need to give those authors' names; this would be a suitable listing in a bibliography; you might have to refer to this source in the unlikely event that you are using material from the preface.

Points to notice: capital *E* for "Eds." (editors), but small *e* for "ed." (edition).

CHAPTER IN EDITED BOOK, THREE AUTHORS

Field, P. A., Stinson, S. M., & Thibaudeau, M-F. (1992). Graduate nursing education in Canada. In A. J. Baumgart & J. Larsen (Eds.), <u>Canadian nursing faces the future</u> (2nd ed.) (pp. 421-445). Toronto: Mosby-Year Book.

In body of paper: (Field, Stinson, & Thibaudeau, 1992); with a quotation: (Field, Stinson, & Thibaudeau, 1992, pp. xx-xx).

Points to notice: commas around initials; the hyphen in Thibaudeau's initials, a convention for a hyphenated first name (Marie-France); position of initials for editors of the book; position of page numbers for the chapter; use of abbreviation pp. when page numbers for the chapter are given; use of separate parentheses around edition number and chapter page numbers.

BOOK REPRINTED FROM ORIGINAL

Nightingale, F. (1946). <u>Notes on nursing: What it is, and what it is not.</u> Philadelphia: Lippincott. (Original work published 1859)

In body of paper: (Nightingale, 1946); with a quotation: (Nightingale, 1946, p. xx). But you should make it clear in the text that the original was published earlier through reference either to this well-known author or to the year the original appeared.

Point to notice: no period at the end of the citation.

BOOK, GROUP OR AGENCY AUTHOR

American Psychological Association. (1994). <u>Publication manual of the American Psychological Association</u> (4th ed.). Washington, DC: Author.

In body of paper: if mentioned only once (American Psychological Association, 1994); with a quotation: (American Psychological Association, 1994, p. xx). If mentioned more than once, use (American Psychological Association [APA], 1994) for the first mention, then (APA, 1994) thereafter. When the group or agency is well known and frequently referred to by its initials (e.g., American Psychological Association [APA], Canadian Nurses Association [CNA], or World Health Organization [WHO]), and you are referring to it often in your paper, use the abbreviation.

Point to notice: postal code designations for provinces, states, and countries are not considered abbreviations and do not need periods.

BOOK, GOVERNMENT AGENCY AS AUTHOR

Statistics Canada. (1981). <u>Standard occupational classification 1980</u> (Catalogue 12-565E). Ottawa: Minister of Supply and Services Canada.

In body of paper: (Statistics Canada, 1981); with a quotation: (Statistics Canada, 1981, p. xx).

Point to notice: many government documents have either catalogue numbers or report numbers, and whenever possible they should be included (if your readers ever need to find the report, this number really helps a librarian track it down).

JOURNAL ARTICLE, ONE AUTHOR, PAGINATED BY VOLUME

Hawley, M. P. (1992). Sources of stress for emergency nurses in four urban Canadian emergency departments. Journal of Emergency Nursing, 18, 211-216.

In body of paper: (Hawley, 1992); with a quotation: (Hawley, 1992, p. xx).

Points to notice: capitals used for all major words in the title of a journal because it represents a proper name; underlining for the title includes the volume number but not the page range.

JOURNAL ARTICLE, ONE AUTHOR, PAGINATED BY ISSUE

Wylie, D. M. (1996). Perspectives on the staff nurse [editorial]. Canadian Journal of Nursing Administration, 9(2), 5-6.

In body of paper: (Wylie, 1996); with a quotation (Wylie, 1996, p. x).

Points to notice: information about a special kind of article (e.g., editorial, letter to the editor) is noted in brackets following the title; no spacing between volume and issue numbers.

JOURNAL ARTICLE, THREE TO FIVE AUTHORS

Cameron, S. J., Keil, J., Rajacich, D., & Dunham, K. (1996). Using functional health patterns to predict outcome with seniors. The Canadian Nurse: L'infirmière canadienne, 92(10), 34-38.

In body of paper: on first mention (Cameron, Keil, Rajacich, & Dunham, 1996); with a quotation: (Cameron, Keil, Rajacich, & Dunham, 1996, p. xx). For subsequent mentions, use (Cameron et al., 1996) or (Cameron et al., 1996, p. xx), unless there is more than one article published in 1996 by a group of authors headed by Cameron. If this happens (albeit rarely in student papers), then you need to list as many authors as necessary to distinguish between the two citations; this number may be two, followed by et al., or it may be the whole list.

Points to notice: use of period in et al.; full name of journal used; note the lack of capitals in the French-language name, which is the way it is used as a proper name by this particular journal.

JOURNAL ARTICLE, SIX OR MORE AUTHORS

Cilistka, D., Mitchell, A., Baumann, A., Sheppard, K., Van Berkel, C., Adam, V., Underwood, J., & Southwell, D. (1996). Changing nursing practice—Trisectoral collaboration in decision making. Canadian Journal of Nursing Administration, 9(2), 60-73.

In body of paper: on first mention (Cilistka et al., 1996); with a quotation: (Cilistka et al., 1996, p. xx), unless there are two or more citations for the same year with Cilistka as the first author. If there are (rare), then list as many authors as necessary, followed by et al., to distinguish between the two full citations.

Points to notice: in the full citation, you list *all* the authors, no matter how many; within the paper, you can shorten the reference using et al.

JOURNAL ARTICLE, NO VOLUME OR ISSUE NUMBER

Bellows, G. (1997, November 14). The culture of flowers. Surrey Horticulture, pp. 21-22, 24.

In body of paper: (Bellows, 1997); with a quotation: (Bellows, 1997, p. xx).

Points to notice: the month is not abbreviated; the abbreviation pp. is used before page numbers; the comma in this page number sequence indicates that the pages are not continuous — that is, the article runs on pages 21 and 22, but something else (maybe an ad) is on page 23, and the article continues and concludes on page 24.

JOURNAL ARTICLE, NO AUTHOR NAMED

The joy of flowers. (1997, November 14). Surrey Horticulture, pp. 11-12, 14.

In body of paper: ("The Joy of Flowers," 1997); with a quotation: ("The Joy of Flowers," 1997, p. xx).

Points to notice: when no author's name is given with an article, it is harder to use the author-year style; when this happens, the first element of the reference is the title; within your paper, you also identify the article by its title, followed by the year; if the title is long, use only a portion of it followed by an ellipsis of three dots, as in the following:

Wildflowers give fields special beauty during autumn months. (1997, November 14). Surrey Horticulture, pp. 16-19.

In body of paper: ("Wildflowers Give Fields ...," 1997); with a quotation: ("Wildflowers Give Fields ...," 1997, p. xx).

VIDEOTAPE OR FILM

British Columbia Nurses' Union. (c1992). As hearts turn (Video). (Available from B.C. Nurses' Union, 100—4259 Canada Way, Burnaby, BC V5G 1H1).

In body of paper: (B.C. Nurses' Union, c1992); it is unlikely that you would use a direct quotation from the film, but if you do you do not need to specify a point on the film; if more than one reference to this video in the paper, use (B.C. Nurses' Union [BCNU], c1992) on first mention and (BCNU, c1992) for subsequent mentions.

Points to notice: abbreviation of British Columbia to B.C., which is suitable if you are writing within Canada for a Canadian audience, but it needs to be spelled out if you are writing for an American journal; use of periods when B.C. is an abbreviation, but not in the postal code designation; use of the apostrophe, which is part of BCNU's proper name; use of c1992, because there is no date given on this tape (the small c stands for circa, which means "about"); use of the full address, although it may not be necessary for some audiences, in which case you would just say (Available from B.C. Nurses' Union).

UNPUBLISHED OR LIMITED-CIRCULATION DOCUMENTS

Zilm, G. (1994). The write way: A distance education work book. Unpublished course material, University of Victoria School of Nursing Distance Education in Nursing Program, Victoria, BC.

In body of paper: (Zilm, 1994); with a quotation: (Zilm, 1994, p. xx).

Points to notice: similar to other unpublished documents such as theses; the city comes after the place where the unpublished material was presented, distributed, or stored.

Bramadat, I. (1995, January). 49:703 Course syllabus: Foundations, issues & trends in nursing. Unpublished course syllabus, University of Manitoba School of Nursing, Winnipeg, MB.

In body of paper: (Bramadat, 1995); in the rare instance that you use a direct quotation from such material: (Bramadat, 1995, p. x).

Points to notice: the punctuation, including the ampersand (&), in the title is copied exactly from the title used in the course syllabus; do not necessarily follow the style you use in your own documents.

MATERIAL FROM A CD-ROM

Tynes, L. L. (1993). Tuberculosis: The continuing story. JAMA: Journal of the American Medical Association, 270, 2616-2617. Text from: InfoTrac Health Reference Center July '92-July '95

In body of paper: (Tynes, 1993); even if you use a direct quotation, you cannot usually give a page number because the file printed out on your printer will be in a different format; it is possible to use (Tynes, 1993, l. xx), with l. standing for "line."

Points to notice: this example is taken from a CD-ROM from a company called the Health Reference Center. It supplies disks monthly to subscribers (e.g., libraries, hospitals, wealthy individuals). Each new disk contains abstracts and sometimes complete texts purchased by this service from more than 300 professional medical and nursing journals and kept on the disk for the most recent three-year period. Readers can browse electronically through all these recent journals using keywords to find relevant articles and may then print out the abstract or, if available, the full text. For the article in this example, you might also obtain the original journal if it is available locally, although in the future much of this kind of material may be published only on CD-ROM or on-line. On some CD-ROMs (although not this one), each item has a file retrieval number; if so, it is given at the end of the item.

ELECTRONIC DATA FILE OR DATABASE

Organization for Economic Co-operation and Development. (1993). Life expectancy and infant mortality: OECD/World Health Organization data 1987-88. OECD health data: Comparative analysis of health systems (Computer file). Paris, France: CREDES File: **-***

In body of paper: (Organization for Economic Co-operation and Development, 1993); even if you use a direct quotation (and it would likely be better to paraphrase), you cannot usually give a page number because the file may have printed out on your printer in a different format; if you use the reference more than once in the paper, indicate the abbreviated form on the first mention (Organization for Economic Co-operation and Development [OECD], 1993) and use (OECD, 1993) for subsequent mentions.

Points to notice: this example is taken from a file accessible to the Manitoba Health Department. CREDES is a Paris-based international information source, to which libraries and some government agencies may subscribe (similar to MEDLINE). Once you have a subscription number (or are a student at a college or university with a subscription to this information source), you can access the document on your computer and then use the file number (deleted here and replaced with asterisks) to find the file. The spelling of "co-operation" (with the hyphen) follows part of the proper name of this organization and thus needs to be copied correctly.

ON-LINE MATERIAL — DRUG REFERENCE

United States Pharmacopeial Convention, Inc. (1994). Imodium (oral). In United States Pharmacopeial Convention, Inc., Consumer Reports complete drug reference (On-line). Available: AOL Reference Desk December 12, 1996

In body of paper: (United States Pharmacopeial Convention, Inc., 1994).

Points to notice: drug reference material can be obtained in a number of ways, including access to a pharmacopoeia maintained in the hospital in which you are working or studying. I obtained a printout of eight single-spaced pages of material after I did a search for information on this drug on my home computer using my America Online (AOL) service. The path I chose was the AOL Reference Desk page; I selected the "Health and Medicine" menu, then used the menu item "Drug References," then clicked on the menu item *"Consumer Reports Complete Drug Reference,"* and finally typed in the name of the drug (keyword "Imodium") to retrieve the material. *Consumer Reports* gets initial capital letters because this is a proper name of a journal; no punctuation is used at the end of the specified path.

MATERIAL FROM AN ON-LINE JOURNAL WITH AUTHOR

Sparkman, R. (1995). For women with severe premenstrual syndrome, antidepressants really can lift the blues — although some worries linger. HEALTH Magazine Online. Available: AOL Newsstand, HEALTH Magazine Online Document ID mrsn95p

In body of paper: (Sparkman, 1995); with a quotation: (Sparkman, 1995, para. **).

Points to notice: this example is taken from an on-line journal that I reached on my home computer using my America Online service. I chose the Newsstand icon from the main menu and then selected *HEALTH Magazine*, selected the Search icon, entered "multivitamins" as a keyword, and received this document as one of two possible items connected to this keyword; note the document ID number, which may make it easier for others to find this document if they have to search through another on-line service. No punctuation is used at the end of the specified path.

MATERIAL FROM AN ON-LINE JOURNAL, NO AUTHOR

Tuberculosis. (1995). HEALTH Magazine Online. Available: AOL Newsstand, HEALTH Magazine Online Document ID tuberc

In body of paper: ("Tuberculosis," 1995); with a quotation: ("Tuberculosis," 1995, l. *-**).

Points to notice: this example is taken from an on-line journal that I reached on my home computer using my America Online service. I chose the Newsstand icon from the main menu and then selected *HEALTH Magazine*, selected the Search icon, entered "tuberculosis" as a keyword, and received this document as one of one possible items connected to this keyword; this is a brief item, likely used to fill up space between articles. It is marked "Copyright Time Publishing Ventures, Inc.," which might indicate that it has been reprinted or abridged from another source; l. stands for line — this item is only 18 lines long.

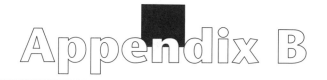

Sample Student Paper

The following pages show portions of a fictional student paper to illustrate one way that you might set up a short and relatively simple paper. Remember, however, that you must think SMART. Different instructors (audience) might ask for different layouts. The information presented in some papers (message) might call for a more complex format. If you are thoroughly familiar with APA style, you (source) might wish to amend this layout slightly to fit with your views about a good presentation.

The following paper was written in response to this fictional request:

Assignment 2 (due December 8, 1998)

Write a brief essay (about 1,500 words or maximum seven pages of text) in which you recommend reference books that would be helpful to first-year nursing students. Use the *Publication Manual of the American Psychological Association* (4th ed.) (APA, 1994) as a guide for formatting your paper. Please supply an outline and table of contents.

THE WRITE TOOLS

by Glennis Zilm
Student Number: 98-7654321

Running head: Write Tools

Assignment #2 (December 8, 1998)
Writing Skills Course E107x
University of Surrey

Instructor: Cheryl Entwistle, RN, BSN, MA

Glennis Zilm
#306 — 1521 Blackwood St.
White Rock, BC V4B 3V6
Phone: 535-3238

Write Tools   2

Table of Contents

The Write Tools: Outline

I. Introduction
  — short section introducing the paper, stating that students need to have good writing tools (called "the write tools") on hand to help them with their courses and giving my recommendations for the best ones

II. Body of Paper
  A. Dictionary
  —

  B. Grammar Book
  —

  C. Style Manual
  — What is a style manual?
  — Why it is needed

III. Conclusion

The Write Tools

Students who hope to do well in their courses need good writing skills. Good writers usually have a shelf of "writing tools" to help them. In particular, students should have three "write tools" on their desks (or on a shelf near the desk): a good dictionary, a basic grammar book, and an approved style manual. In this paper, I give a brief outline of each of these tools and why each is useful. I also recommend the ones I believe students should own.

Dictionary

A good, college-level dictionary is an essential tool for any student writer — even if he or she uses a computer that has a spell checker built in. Dictionaries are much more than lists of words spelled correctly. They provide information on shades of meaning of synonyms (e.g., character, personality, individuality). They offer information on pronunciation of words (e.g., various pronunciations of lever). They point out distinctions in homographs, which are words that sound the same but have different spellings and different meanings (e.g., root, route), and homonyms, which are words that are spelled and sound the same but have different meanings (e.g., rose [flower], rose [past tense of rise]). They distinguish between various tones of meaning (e.g., formal, informal, slang, derogatory, archaic). They provide valuable information on how a word is used (e.g., as a noun or verb or both). They may even provide information on the origins of the word and the changes it has gone through during its history.

Dictionaries often reflect the country of origin, such as those written and published in Britain or in the United States. Canadian students likely should own a Canadian dictionary, although some colleges recommend use of a specific dictionary. The Gage Canadian Dictionary (de Wolf, Gregg, Harris, & Scargill, 1997) is my personal choice. It was originally compiled in 1983 by a group of five distinguished Canadian lexicographers and has been revised and brought up to date to reflect current Canadian usage. The original 1983 dictionary contains a wonderful essay on "Canadian English" by Professor Walter S. Avis; it makes one proud of Canadian English for its depth and breadth. Although this essay is not included in the recent revision, the introductory section contains a good summary of it.

Grammar Book

Even students who feel reasonably secure about their writing skills will benefit by having a sound grammar book among their write tools....

References and Bibliography

American Psychological Association. (1994). <u>Publication manual of the American Psychological Association</u> (4th ed.). Washington, DC: Author.

Avis, W. S., Drysdale, P. D., Gregg, R. J., Neufeldt, V. E., & Scargill, M. H. (Compilers). (1983). <u>Gage Canadian dictionary.</u> Toronto: Gage.

Buckley, J. (1995). <u>Fit to print: The Canadian student's guide to essay writing</u> (3rd ed.). Toronto: Harcourt Brace Canada.

Day, R. A. (1988). <u>How to write and publish a scientific paper</u> (3rd ed.). Phoenix: Oryx Press.

de Wolf, G. D., Gregg, R. J., Harris, B. P., & Scargill, M. H. (Compilers). (1997). <u>Gage Canadian dictionary</u> (rev.). Toronto: Gage.

Entwistle, C. (1998). <u>E107x Course Syllabus, University of Surrey Department of English.</u> Surrey, BC: University of Surrey Department of English.

Northey, M., & Timney, B. (1995). <u>Making sense in psychology and the life sciences: A student's guide to writing and style.</u> Toronto: Oxford University Press.

. . . .

Note: The reference for the *Gage Canadian Dictionary* could be done in several ways. Usually, dictionaries are put into reference lists using this style:

<u>Gage Canadian dictionary</u>. (1983). Toronto: Gage.

However, because there are now two editions and because I wanted to refer to an essay by one of the compilers in the paper, I used the longer version.

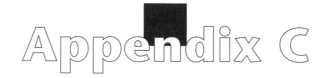

Appendix C

Sample Business Communications for Nurses

This section contains sample business communications illustrating layouts and offering some ideas that might be adapted depending on Source * Message * Audience * Route * Tone.

Sample Letter of Application for a Job
Sample Query Letter to a Journal
Sample Covering Letter
Sample Letter to the Editor
Sample Short Progress Report (Memo Format)

All information in these communications is fictional and is designed to illustrate layout and writing skills. The messages are not intended to represent actual situations.

SAMPLE LETTER OF APPLICATION FOR A JOB

1234 Urban Street
Thunder Bay, AB   T8G 0X0

June 23, 1997

Human Resources/Personnel Office
Well Known Regional Hospital
4321 Main Street
Prince George, BC   V2L 0N0

RE: Application for Registered Nurse Position

My husband and I are moving to Prince George in mid-August, and I am seeking a position as a staff nurse. He will be joining the teaching staff at Prince George Elementary School.

As you will see from my résumé, I graduated in late April from the School of Nursing at Thunder Bay Community College, and I have passed my Registered Nurse exams. I am registered with the Alberta Association of Registered Nurses, and I applied for registration with the Registered Nurses Association of B.C. earlier this month.

Since graduation, I have been working as a casual relief nurse at the Eagle Ridge Hospital near Thunder Bay, mainly in the Long Term Care Units. The local hospitals do not have any openings for full-time staff, but I have been assured that my work skills are excellent, and I would be in line for a full-time position should one arise. My unit supervisors have agreed to supply letters if you require references. As well as my nursing jobs, I have worked part-time as an assistant in a day care centre (12 infants).

I would like to receive information about your hospital and application forms for a possible RN position. If you expect to have an opening before mid-August and would like to discuss it with me, I can be reached by telephone at (403) 555-2112.

Sincerely

(Mrs.) Geraldine Summers, RN

Points to note

Jobs for new graduates are extremely scarce in Canada in the late 1990s. This preliminary letter, sent before a move to a new location, should elicit application forms and some information about the hospital and its human relations department (perhaps including the name of the person who receives the applications for RN positions).

SAMPLE QUERY LETTER TO A JOURNAL

ANNE AUTHOR, RN, BSN

1357 Broad Avenue
Black Tusk, SK S0G 1X7

Phone (306) 555-9876
E-mail aauthor@bol.com

January 6, 1997

Judith Raines, Editor-in-Chief
The National Nurse
50 Broadway
Ottawa, ON   K2P 0Y0

Dear Ms Raines

RE: Query Concerning Submission of Manuscript

Despite increased knowledge about infectious diseases and the success of early treatment, pneumonia remains in third place as the killer of children under one year of age. Only congenital anomalies/birth defects and neonatal accidents rank higher. Nurses have a major role to play in educating parents about the high incidence of pneumonia in babies, its rapid onset in young infants, its early signs and symptoms, and its prevention.

Last summer two colleagues and I carried out a small research project on pneumonia in early childhood in our local area and on the role that nurses can play in reducing the incidence. We interviewed 65 mothers living in our region whose children had been diagnosed with pneumonia to discover how it might have been prevented or reduced in severity. Our findings show that information from nurses could serve as a first line of defence.

Would you be interested in reviewing an article on this topic for possible publication? Our study contains specific recommendations for public health nurses, nurses in doctors' offices, and neonatal nurses. However, we found that mothers often seek advice from any nurses they know during the early stages of the baby's "cold" and that all nurses need to be more aware of the dangers of pneumonia in early childhood. The comments from the families on the kind of assistance needed from nurses are interesting. We believe most readers of *The National Nurse* would find the article of interest.

I am a community nurse with the Cypress Hills Regional Health District in southern Saskatchewan. Beth Second is a nurse in a pediatrician's office, and Mary Third is the head nurse of the pediatric unit at Cypress District Hospital. Our study was supported by the Regional Health District's Nursing Research Fund. We have completed and submitted a report to the funding agency. We would be able to provide you with an article of about 2,000 words, if you are interested, and could complete the article by early spring.

I look forward to hearing from you about your possible interest and would welcome any comments and suggestions you may have.

Sincerely

(Miss) Anne Author, RN, BSN

Points to note

Although this letter is a little long, it offers considerable detail that would enable the editor to judge the merits of a possible manuscript. For example, the opening is intended to arouse interest and show that the author(s) can take a creative approach rather than begin with the trite opening "Would you be interested in reviewing an article on pneumonia in infants?"

This letter, like most other good business letters, covers who, what, when, where, why, and how.

This letter shows that the writer has considered the potential readers of the journal; the majority of readers of *The National Nurse* are hospital staff nurses rather than community health nurses or pediatric nurses. So Anne Author mentions that mothers ask "any nurses they know" — which means that almost all nurses who receive this journal would benefit from reading this article. As well, the writer shows that she has read the "Information for Authors" page that is published regularly in this journal, because the length suggested is what the editors request.

This letter gives enough background about the authors so that the editor can judge if they would be a good source for information on the subject.

SAMPLE COVERING LETTER

ANNE AUTHOR, RN, BSN

1357 Broad Avenue   Phone (306) 555-9876
Black Tusk, SK S0G 1X7   E-mail aauthor@bol.com

March 25, 1997

Judith Raines, Editor-in-Chief
The National Nurse
50 Broadway
Ottawa, ON K2P 0Y0

Dear Judith Raines

   Attached are three copies of our manuscript "Pneumonia in Newborns," by Anne Author, Beth Second, and Mary Third. I wrote to you about this article in early January, and you expressed interest in reviewing it for possible publication in *The National Nurse*.

   The article runs about 1,960 words and is based on the research study we carried out last fall. The article describes roles that nurses can play in educating and advising mothers so that the incidence of this childhood killer may be reduced. I have also enclosed a page giving background information on the authors and a note acknowledging funding from the Cypress Hills Regional Health District's Nursing Research Fund. As well, there is a signed statement from all three authors acknowledging the submission of this article.

   If you are interested, I may be able to supply a few posed photographs to illustrate the article. Our health unit strongly supported this project, and the photos were taken for the local newspaper when the project was being carried out.

   I hope you will decide to accept the article for publication. I look forward to hearing from you.

                                   Sincerely

Points to note

This covering letter not only ensures that the article is directed to the appropriate individual but also provides additional information about other enclosures and about the possible photographs. However, it is still short and to the point.

SAMPLE LETTER TO THE EDITOR
(COVER LETTER FIRST)

7135 Narrows Street
White Tusk, NS B1K 0X0

March 25, 1997

Judith Raines, Editor-in-Chief
The National Nurse
50 Broadway
Ottawa, ON   K2P 0Y0

Dear Ms Raines

   I hope *The National Nurse* will consider publishing the attached letter to the editor.

   If you have any questions or concerns, you can reach me at my home number (902 - 555-8776); early evenings are the best time to reach me. You can also leave a message for me on e-mail at a&r_onymous@bol.com.

Sincerely

Ann Onymous (Mrs. R. K.)
Third-year student
Balhousie University School of Nursing

Points to note

Letters to the editor need to be formatted so that they can be handled like a manuscript and sent for typesetting. As well, a published letter in a professional journal usually does not contain a street address, only the city; a covering letter giving address, phone number, and other relevant details is therefore attached to the typescript for the letter to be considered for publication.

A Staff-and-Student Networking Idea

Opportunities for nursing students to network with practising registered nurses are vital but seem to be difficult to set up. However, RNs at Seal Cove District Hospital near Halifax, Nova Scotia, have involved students from the Balhousie Nursing Program in small, informal, practical network groups in a way that benefits both nurses and students.

For several years, staff nurses from the pediatric unit regularly met informally over coffee in the hospital cafeteria for one hour at the end of the day shift every other Thursday to exchange information on current nursing literature. Those who participated took turns reviewing current journals in the hospital's staff library and reporting to the group on articles of interest. Not all staff could attend every time, but several staff found the sessions valuable, and the meetings settled into a routine. The one-hour time limit was strictly observed.

About one year ago, these pediatric nurses invited students assigned to the ward to attend the meetings. The students proved enthusiastic participants, and some asked if they could continue to drop in after they finished the ward assignment. The staff nurses agreed, and the reading group has become larger, with three students interested in pursuing pediatric nursing becoming regular participants. These students have access through the university library to pediatric journals not regularly received in the hospital, and this access benefits the staff group. Students benefit from the regular friendly contact with practising nurses and from hearing practical discussions related to the literature.

Furthermore, the students have reported the idea in other departments, and two other "reading groups" have been set up at Seal Cove Hospital, one by nurses in the emergency department, and one by the geriatric staff; several students from Balhousie take part regularly. Nursing administration at the hospital has supported this informal continuing education project by supplying free coffee, tea, or juice for meetings of all three groups.

The Boundary Health Unit in Seal Cove also has set up a "Literary Lunch Bunch" and invites students assigned to the unit to take part. Unfortunately, few students can continue this involvement once the community health assignment is over, because the midday time conflicts with class schedules. At least one student, however, has been an off-and-on regular with this group for six months and now plans to follow a career in public health.

Nurses who participate in reading groups in other parts of Canada might want to consider including students. I know from experience that this form of networking is much appreciated.

Ann Onymous
Third-year student, Balhousie University
White Tusk, NS

More points to note

The typescript of a letter to the editor (or other possible item sent to a journal, such as a news item, book review, or classified ad) should be double spaced, with typical wide margins and each page clearly labelled with a running head and the page number. Follow the style guide required by the journal. You do not need to have a title page for a letter to the editor; the covering letter takes on this role for short items that probably will not be sent for peer review.

Note the short paragraphs, which make reading easier. Letters in journals or newspapers are usually set in narrow columns, and even a short paragraph will look long in such a column.

Letters to the editor are one of the most popular sections in any journal and get the attention of a lot of readers. If you can keep your message relatively short (as in the 420-word letter above), it will likely attract more readers than will an article on the same subject.

The section for Letters to the Editor frequently has a word limit (often with a maximum word count of 450 words); check the beginning and end of the section in the journal to see if length is mentioned. Even if the journal does not specify length, keep the letter as short as possible; it is then more likely to be accepted for publication.

SAMPLE SHORT PROGRESS REPORT (MEMO FORMAT)

Well Known Hospital
54321 Major Drive
Well Known City, BC   V4Z X0O

TO: Jane Doe, Vice-President Patient Services

FROM: John Singh, RN, Unit Manager OR   PHONE: local 123

DATE: 16 March 1997

RE: Progress Report on WKH Auxiliary Special Funding

The Operating Room received a one-time special grant of $13,000 from the WKH Auxiliary in December 1996 to purchase operating room instruments. The purchase is progressing on time and on budget, with instruments worth $11,769 (including relevant taxes, delivery, and so on) ordered and received. When one more back order is received, the rest of the money will have been used.

Background

At a meeting of WKH OR staff, a list was drawn up of instruments often requested by surgeons but unavailable or in short supply. These instruments were in addition to those requested in the 1996-1997 OR budget; some items that had to be cut from the budget were included in this list.

OR staff then prepared a proposal for funding, in consultation with the Materiels Manager. The proposal was supported by the WKH Medical Committee and approved by WKH Administration. The funding proposal was submitted to the WKH Auxiliary in November, and the Auxiliary approved the $13,000 request at its meeting in early December.

The list included
- instruments for specialty work in ear surgery now that this specialty surgery is available at WKH;
- additional basic instruments to help shorten turn-around times for operations.

Orders to Date

On 13 January 1997, three magnifying lenses and a complete set of auricular instruments, including pinna scrapers, antihelix retractors, ossicle retrievers, and tympani forceps, were ordered from Ear-Ache Instruments of Toronto. These instruments arrived 12 February 1997. One of the magnifying lenses was scratched on arrival and has been returned; a replacement is on its way. All other instruments were checked and incorporated into OR stocks. Total cost of these instruments was $10,343.

A list of 12 special retractors often requested by surgeons was drawn up by OR staff and checked with the Chief of Surgery. The order was placed 19 January 1997 with Retractor-Magic of Montreal and received 19 February. Total cost was $1,426.

An OR micro-sterilizer for auricular instruments has been ordered through 3X Instruments of Boston (there is no Canadian supplier). The list price is $987 (US); this should use most of the remaining funds but remain within the funding budget. Expected date of delivery is 20 March 1997. Final cost will depend on the exchange rate when the order is received. If the cost exceeds the $13,000 grant, the few extra dollars will be taken from the general OR budget for supplies.

Copies of the purchase orders for all items, with prices, are attached for information.

<u>Future Actions</u>

All equipment should be received and in use by 5 April 1997.

Once all equipment is received and put into use, letters from the OR Head Nurse, the Chief of Surgery, and the new ENT Specialist will be written and sent to the WKH Auxiliary President outlining the use and thanking members for the grant.

Copy: J. Hancock, Materiels Manager

JS/sac

Points to note

A memo format was used for this response to a request for a (written) progress report on the use of the Auxiliary's money. Although it is only two pages long, it still likely tells Jane Doe more than she needs to know. However, it provides all the information that she may need if she has to discuss the matter with the Auxiliary president — or for whatever other reason that she wanted a written progress report (and not just a quick reply over the telephone). It even includes some review material to help remind her of the background.

Although it uses a long (8.5" x 11") memo form (which tends to make it somewhat informal in tone), John Singh arranged to have it typed for him (note the typist's initials), which makes it more formal. Furthermore, the typed version fits onto two pages; a handwritten version would likely require more pages. As well, the language and the writing style tend to be formal.

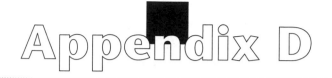

Annotated Bibliography: Useful Readings/ Reference Tools

This annotated bibliography identifies books that I used in compiling this text and provides information on useful readings and good reference tools for nurses who write. You would likely find most of the books mentioned in the "Writing and References" section of a college or university bookstore. Some seem rather old (e.g., Strunk and White, 1979) but are classics still in print and used in writing courses. In some instances, you may find a later edition than the one mentioned here.

The style used in this list differs from the style recommended in the fourth edition of the *Publication Manual of the American Psychological Association* (APA, 1994). APA style was used for the references at the end of each chapter. The style used in this bibliography is based on the style recommended in *Webster's Standard American Style Guide* (1985). *Webster's* style is the one most commonly used in books written for general readers (audience); APA style is used for social science and health care scientific writing (a different audience). *Webster's* recommends use of capital letters in book titles (other style guides, including APA, do not), and the year of publication is the final item in the citation. The format is different from APA as well; *Webster's* recommends use of a "hanging indent" in which the second and subsequent lines are indented so that the authors' names are more obvious.

I prefer *Webster's* style for bibliographic lists. I also like to know the first names of authors and include them in my own lists; most style guides do not recommend the use of the full first names, but as a source I can decide to use them in my book (route), provided my publisher allows this approach. I find this modified style well suited to annotated bibliographies and reading lists (message). If I write for a journal, I follow its style, of course. The full-name style takes quite a bit more space, so it is not suitable for most research journals. I have tried to make the tone used in the annotations informal so that my readers will not think they must have all these books on their own shelves.

I hope that you will find this list useful when you select your reference tools.

American Psychological Association. *Publication Manual of the American Psychological Association* (4th ed.). Washington, DC: American Psychological Association, 1994.
The most useful style guide for nurses. Buy a copy for your reference shelves as soon as you can afford one.

Avis, W.S., Drysdale, P.D., Gregg, R.J., Neufeldt, V.E., & Scargill, M.H. *Gage Canadian Dictionary.* Toronto: Gage, 1983.
Excellent dictionary for Canadian students at the postsecondary level. A later edition (see de Wolf, Gregg, Harris, & Scargill, 1997, listed below) is available, but the first edition has an excellent introduction to the reasons why a *Canadian* dictionary is important. You must have a good dictionary on your reference shelf (even if you have a spell checker in your computer).

Bell, Louise. *Effective Writing: A Guide for Health Professionals.* Toronto: Copp Clark, 1995.
A good Canadian text for graduate nurses and other health professionals, and one you may wish to add to your reference shelf later in your career. In addition to a more thorough review of grammar, punctuation, and other writing problems, it concentrates on research papers, articles for publication, and health education materials.

Bernstein, Theodore M. *The Careful Writer: A Modern Guide to English Usage.* New York: Atheneum, 1973.
An old book, recently reissued. A useful reference if you tend to misuse words.

Bernstein, Theodore M. *Miss Thistlebottom's Hobgoblins: The Careful Writer's Guide to the Taboos, Bugbears and Out-Moded Rules of English Usage*. New York: Farrar, Straus and Giroux, 1971.

A delightful book by a master writer; it reports on changes in English grammar, punctuation, and style. If you like writing and words, and can find this or any of Bernstein's books (now out of print) in a library, then borrow and savor them. Look for them in second-hand bookstores if you are interested in the English language.

Birch, Ann. *Essay Writing Made Easy: Presenting Ideas in All Subject Areas*. Markham, ON: Pembroke Publishers, 1993.

An excellent little book. Offers suggestions for researching your topic — especially "limiting your topic" — and for drawing on your own experiences and interviewing experts (personal communications).

Buckley, J. *Fit to Print: The Canadian Student's Guide to Essay Writing* (3rd ed.). Toronto: Harcourt Brace Canada, 1995.

Excellent reference tool covering much the same ground as this text but with more detail on essay writing for arts courses, such as English, and with more emphasis on errors of grammar and punctuation.

Chicago Guide to Preparing Electronic Manuscripts for Authors and Publishers. Chicago: University of Chicago Press, 1987.

Useful when you progress to the point in your career where you have to submit an electronic manuscript of a book to a publisher, but otherwise fairly esoteric. Check for later editions, because the technology is constantly changing.

The Chicago Manual of Style (14th ed.). Chicago: University of Chicago Press, 1993.

The classic style manual that forms the basis for style by most book publishers; the first edition, published in 1906, was one of the first style guides.

Council of Biology Editors. *Scientific Style and Format: The CBE Manual for Authors, Editors, and Publishers* (6th ed.). New York: Cambridge University Press, 1994.

Another big style manual of the same genre as the APA manual. Borrow it if you are writing for a journal that uses CBE style.

Council of Biology Editors. *Scientific Writing for Graduate Students: A Manual on the Teaching of Scientific Writing*. Bethesda, MD: Author, 1986.

If you are going into a master's or doctoral program, you should at least review a copy of this manual. Old but still an excellent reference tool for graduate students. A new edition is being considered.

Cremmins, Edward T. *The Art of Abstracting*. Philadelphia: iSi Press, 1982.

A whole book on how to write an abstract! You probably should borrow it from a library when you come to work on the abstract for your master's thesis or doctoral dissertation.

Davies, Barbara, & Logan, Jo. *Reading Research: A User-Friendly Guide for Nurses and Other Health Care Professionals*. Ottawa: Canadian Nurses Association, 1993.

An excellent guide for students just entering a nursing program on how to read, understand, and evaluate the quality of research articles published in professional journals. Although this small, inexpensive pamphlet is directed toward readers of research articles, you can also deduce many applications for you as a writer.

Day, Robert A. *Scientific English: A Guide for Scientists and Other Professionals* (2nd ed.). Phoenix: Oryx Press, 1995.

An excellent reference tool for those in the final years of a university course or those in graduate school. (The first edition, 1992, might be available in second-hand stores and is just as useful for nurses.)

Day, Robert A. *How to Write and Publish a Scientific Paper* (4th ed.). Phoenix: Oryx Press, 1993.

An excellent book to own if you really like to write and essential if you are taking a master's degree; otherwise, consider borrowing it from a library.

Dittrick, Mark, & Dittrick, Diane Kender. *No Uncertain Terms*. New York: Facts on File Publications, 1984.

Out of print, but a wonderful, witty book that tells you in memorable ways about fine distinctions in meaning between words (e.g., *sweet potato* and *yam*, or *cement* and *concrete*). If you find it in a library, borrow it and browse.

de Wolf, G.D., Gregg, R.J., Harris, B.P., & Scargill, M.H. *Gage Canadian Dictionary* (rev.). Toronto: Gage, 1997.

The most recent edition of a good Canadian dictionary. I recommend this as the best dictionary for your bookshelf.

Dupuis, K. Carew, & Wilson, S.V. *Communicating with P.O.W.E.R.* Toronto: Gage Publishing, 1982.

Old, and my text covers the same basic material, but Dupuis and Wilson provide another way to approach the writing PROCESS.

Elbow, Peter. *Writing with Power: Techniques for Mastering the Writing Process*. New York: Oxford University Press, 1981.

An excellent book if you are already a good writer and want to be even better. Available in most college and university bookstores and recommended in many English departments.

Furberg, Jon, & Hopkins, Richard. *College Style Sheet* (4th ed.). Vancouver: 49th Avenue Press (Langara College), 1996.

This slim, inexpensive volume provides a summary of important points of APA style (but based on the *third* edition) as well as brief explanations of most other style guides used at college and university levels. It also provides excellent sample layouts for typing your papers.

Gordon, Karen Elizabeth. *The Transitive Vampire: A Handbook of Grammar for the Innocent, the Eager, and the Doomed*. New York: Times Books, 1984.

A fun but sound grammar book; the examples are thoroughly modern. If you are having basic problems, however, then Northey and Timney will be more valuable to you.

Gordon, Karen Elizabeth. *The Well-Tempered Sentence: A Punctuation Handbook for the Innocent, the Eager, and the Doomed*. New York: Ticknor & Fields, 1983.

Another fun reference with unique and memorable examples of punctuation errors, with advice on solutions.

Harbert, E.N., & DiGaetani, J.L. *Writing for Action: A Guide for the Health Care Professional*. Homewood, IL: Dow Jones-Irwin, 1984.

Out of print, but a terrific book for those who write at work. Not really applicable for students. Check libraries and try to borrow a copy if you work in a hospital and have to write reports.

Li, Xia, & Crane, Nancy B. *Electronic Style: A Guide to Citing Electronic Information*. Westport, CT: Mecklermedia, 1993.

A small, expensive book that may be useful to graduate students using many electronic documents in literature reviews and thesis preparation. Needs updating.

MacLennan, Jennifer. *Effective Business Writing* (2nd ed.). Scarborough, ON: Prentice-Hall Canada, 1995.

A basic book on letters, memos, reports, and résumés, with many examples showing formats. Also contains useful general comments on ways to develop a clear, concise, complete, and courteous business writing style.

McFarlane, J.A., & Clements, Warren. *The Globe and Mail Style Book*. Toronto: Info Globe, 1990.

If you plan to write letters to the editor, you need this book. Borrow it from a library and browse in it if you have "letters to the editor" as an assignment. Essential for your reference shelf if you routinely write articles for publication.

Merriam-Webster Dictionary of English Usage. Springfield, MA: Merriam-Webster, 1989.

This basic reference book on English usage is arranged like a dictionary. In many instances, it may tell you more than you wish to know about a subject, but it is perhaps the most useful modern manual on distinctions in usage, although it is decidedly American. If you are an advanced student, you may want it, but a good dictionary — one that explains distinctions in usage — will be suitable for most students.

Miller, Casey, & Swift, Kate. *The Handbook of Nonsexist Writing* (2nd ed.). New York: Harper & Row, 1988.

You will be surprised how much you will learn by reading this book, but the pages on gender bias in the APA (1994) *Manual* are sufficient for most student writers.

Mirin, Susan Kooperstein. *The Nurse's Guide to Writing for Publication.* Wakefield, MA: Nursing Resources/Concept Development, 1981.

Old but available in many nursing libraries. If you plan to write journal articles, this is one of the best guides there is for nurses — but also apply the SMART principles. It contains excellent information on and examples of query letters.

Nemiroff, Greta Hoffman. *Transitions: Succeeding in College and University.* Toronto: Harcourt Brace Canada, 1994.

Written for students, this book gives information on anticipating and solving problems that occur during the difficult transition to the postsecondary student lifestyle (e.g., finance, living quarters, study skills, health). Deals not with writing skills but with lifestyle challenges, which often affect your ability to sit down and get started writing.

Northey, Margot, & Timney, Brian. *Making Sense in Psychology and the Life Sciences: A Student's Guide to Writing and Style* (2nd ed.). Toronto: Oxford University Press, 1995.

Similar to this text, and a relatively good guide for nursing students. Recommended if you continue to have difficulty with the basic organization of paragraphs and essays. Emphasizes preparation of lab reports (e.g., as used in biology or chemistry) and provides excellent examples of grammar and punctuation errors.

Rockowitz, Murray, Brownstein, Samuel C., Hughes, Andrew S., & Peters, Max. *How to Prepare for the GED High School Equivalency Examination: Canadian Edition*. Hauppauge, NY: Barron's Educational Series Inc., 1992. [Various later American editions are available.]

Contains the best review of grammar if you are having basic problems (i.e., if you forget what you learned in grade school). If you are having trouble with the English test required for admission to some colleges and universities, then this is the book for you. As well, any writer would benefit from reviewing the two excellent sections on writing skills. Available in most libraries, including public libraries.

Roman, Kenneth, & Raphaelson, Joel. *Writing That Works: How to Improve Your Memos, Letters, Reports, Speeches, Resumes, Plans, and Other Business Papers* (2nd ed.). New York: HarperPaperbacks, 1992.

A practical pocketbook that can be helpful with business communications, but think SMART to make it really helpful in health care agencies.

Safire, William. *Fumblerules: A Lighthearted Guide to Grammar and Good Usage*. New York: Doubleday, 1990.

A fun grammar book — if you already know your grammar! — and a wonderful book to browse through to review grammar. (Example from page 79: "Never use a long word when a diminutive one will do.")

Sheridan, Donna R., & Dowdney, Donna L. *How to Write and Publish Articles in Nursing*. New York: Springer, 1986.

Old, but such texts no longer seem to be published. You will probably find it in a university or college library. Valuable for students who are good writers and who want to publish while still in the nursing program.

Shertzer, Margaret D. *The Elements of Grammar*. New York: Collier Books/Macmillan Publishing, 1986.

Sound basic grammar book. You may find this one, or one of the earlier editions, on the bookshelves at home.

Strunk, William, Jr., & White, E.B. *The Elements of Style* (3rd ed.). New York: Macmillan, 1979. [Later printings, up to 1996, are available.]

Buy this one. Check second-hand stores to save money, but buy this small classic. It is recommended by the authors of almost every resource in this list. Read it from cover to cover.

Turabian, Kate L. *A Manual for Writers of Term Papers, Theses, and Dissertations* (5th ed.). Chicago: University of Chicago Press, 1987.

A basic style manual. It used to be the standard style guide for arts courses at universities, and some departments still recommend its use.

Vipond, Douglas. *Success in Psychology: Writing and Research for Canadian Students*. Toronto: Harcourt Brace Canada, 1996.
Somewhat similar to this text but for students majoring in psychology. It contains an excellent section on "Working the Library" and another on preparing poster presentations, a special kind of communication.

Webster's Standard American Style Guide. Springfield, MA: Merriam-Webster, 1985.
A general style guide, and an excellent one, although not really applicable to nursing papers. Borrow it from a library and browse through it if you have time.

Zinsser, William. *On Writing Well: An Informal Guide to Writing Nonfiction* (4th ed.). New York: Harper Perennial, 1990.
A classic book about writing — recommended in most university English courses.

INDEX

Reader Reply Card

We are interested in your reaction to *The SMART Way: Writing Skills for Nurses*, by Glennis Zilm. You can help us to improve this book in future editions by completing this questionnaire.

1. What was your reason for using this book?

    ❏ university course ❏ college course ❏ continuing education course

    ❏ professional development ❏ personal interest ❏ other_____

    _____

2. If you are a student, please identify your school and the course in which you used this book.

3. Which chapters or parts of this book did you use? Which did you omit?

4. What did you like best about this book? What did you like least?

5. Please identify any topics you think should be added to future editions.

6. Please add any comments or suggestions.

7. May we contact you for further information?

    Name:_____

    Address: _____

    _____

    Phone: _____

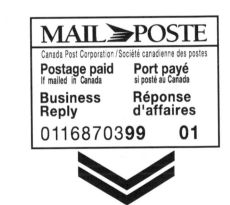

MAIL ➤ POSTE

Canada Post Corporation / Société canadienne des postes

Postage paid **Port payé**
If mailed in Canada si posté au Canada

Business **Réponse**
Reply **d'affaires**

0116870399   01

0116870399-M8Z4X6-BR01

Larry Gillevet
Director of Product Development
HARCOURT BRACE & COMPANY, CANADA
55 HORNER AVENUE
TORONTO, ONTARIO
M8Z 9Z9